A colour atlas of

E. N. T. Diagnosis

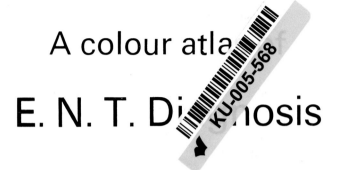

T. R. BULL
F.R.C.S.
Consultant Surgeon
Royal National Throat, Nose and Ear Hospital, London
Lecturer to the Institute of Laryngology and Otology, London
Consultant Surgeon
Metropolitan Ear, Nose and Throat Hospital, London

WOLFE MEDICAL PUBLICATIONS LTD

CONTENTS

UHSM, WYTHENSHAWE
LIBRARY

S221

WV 17 BUL
616.212075

A COLOUR ATLAS OF
E.N.T. DIAGNOSIS

Copyright © T R Bull 1974
Published by Wolfe Medical Publications Ltd 1974
Printed by Smeets-Weert Holland
SBN 7234-0179-9
4th Impression 1979
General Editor, Wolfe Medical Books
G Barry Carruthers MD (Lond)

This book is one of the titles in the series of
Wolfe Medical Atlases, a series which brings
together probably the world's largest systematic
published collection of diagnostic colour
photographs.

For a full list of Atlases in the series, plus
forthcoming titles and details of our surgical,
dental and veterinary Atlases, please write to
Wolfe Medical Publications Ltd.,
Wolfe House, 3-5 Conway Street, London W1P 6HE

ACKNOWLEDGEMENTS

I would like to thank Miss Joselen Ransome, Dr John Hutton, Dr Thomas King, Dr Owen Lloyd and Dr Lamberty for their advice on the text and content of this book. I am also grateful to Mr Connolly of the Institute of Laryngology and Otology and Mr Jaffe of the Metropolitan Ear, Nose and Throat Hospital for their expert help and advice as medical photographers, and to my secretary, Miss Rosemary Fison, for compiling the index.

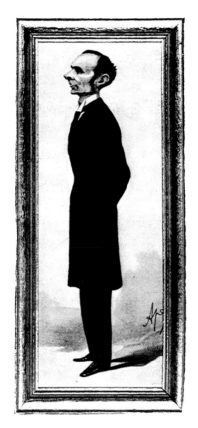

SIR MORRELL MACKENZIE

THIS CARTOON drawn in 1887 shows the austere Scottish physician and surgeon, who founded Ear, Nose and Throat as a speciality and wrote the first standard textbook on Rhinology and Laryngology. Sir Morrell MacKenzie also founded one of the first hospitals for Nose and Throat diseases in London in 1863. The most common condition he treated in this hospital was laryngeal tuberculosis, at that time invariably fatal, and today rare and curable.

Introduction

THIS ATLAS intends to give a pictorial synopsis of Ear, Nose and Throat diseases. Most of the speciality is covered, but there may be a bias towards the conditions that lend themselves to photography. I have tried to avoid too many pictures of gross or excessively obvious pathology so that fairly typical examples of common conditions are shown. Some rareties are included, particularly when they are relevant in the differential diagnosis. Photographs and diagrams of some operations are included for those not familiar wth E.N.T. surgery. Many of the photographs were taken by myself during busy out-patient and operating sessions, and the standard of picture is not uniform: the instruments and technique required to demonstrate the upper respiratory tract and ear make direct referral to the photographic department impractical.

I hope that colour photographs will prove a greater practical help in recognising E.N.T. conditions than drawings or diagrams. This Atlas will, I hope, stimulate an interest in E.N.T. for medical students, and be useful to those in General Practice, Casualty and those training in E.N.T. surgery or allied specialities. A resumé of most conditions is given, but I have made this dogmatic, with no discussion of varying opinions. This Atlas is, therefore, an introduction to Ear, Nose and Throat surgery and an adjunct to the standard textbooks.

Examination

1 The instruments needed for an E.N.T. examination The *head mirror* gives effective lighting for examining the upper respiratory tract and ear, and leaves both hands free for using instruments. Initially, the technique of using a head mirror is not easy.

The *laryngeal and post-nasal mirrors* require warming to avoid misting, and hot water or a spirit lamp is necessary.

An angled *tongue depressor* or wooden spatula is needed for examining the oropharynx and post-nasal space.

Angled forceps are used for dressing the nose or ear.

A *tuning fork* is essential for the diagnosis of conductive deafness or perceptive deafness. A C_1 or C_2 (256 or 512 c.p.s.) is needed. The very large tuning forks to test vibration sense are unsatisfactory and may give a false Rinne test.

A *Jobson-Horne probe* is widely used in E.N.T. departments: a loop on one end is for removing wax (and foreign bodies) from the ear or nose. Cotton wool attached to the other end is used for cleaning the ear.

An *auriscope, nasal and aural specula* complete the basic instruments.

1

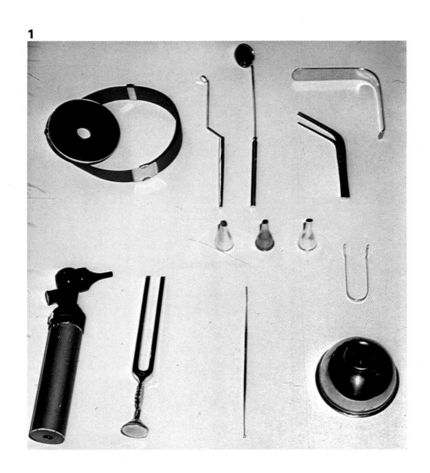

EXAMINATION OF THE EAR

2 Retracting the pinna The meatus is tortuous: to see the drum the pinna is therefore retracted backwards and outwards, and the index finger may be used to hold the tragus forward.

3 The auriscope This is best held like a pen. In this way, the examiner's little finger can rest on the patient's cheek; if the patient's head moves, the position of the ear speculum is maintained in the meatus.

4 Head mirror and speculum These are used for the initial examination of the meatus and drum.

5 A Siegle's speculum This can be attached to magnify the drum, and air is inflated to test the drum's mobility. Normally the drum moves readily, but if the movement is sluggish or absent it suggests middle ear fluid or a thick scarred drum, which may be adherent to the promontory.

2

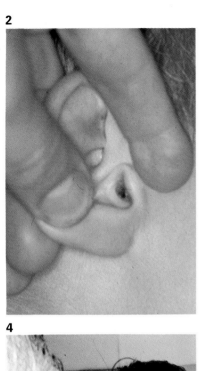

3

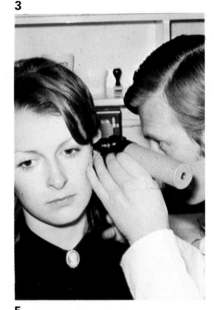

4

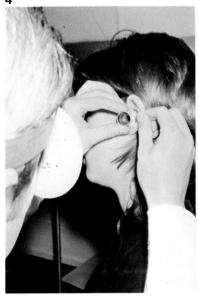

5

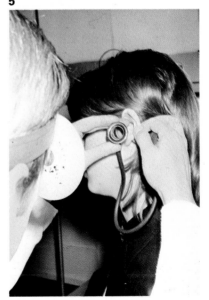

11

The tympanic membrane is grey and translucent.

6   A normal drum   The main landmarks seen on the pars tensa of a normal drum are the short process (*top arrow*) and handle (*middle arrow*) of the malleus and the light reflex (*lower arrow*). The drum superior to the short process is the pars flaccida or attic part of the drum. A normal drum varies in vascularity and translucency.

7   A more vascular drum with vessels extending down the handle of the malleus to the umbo.

8   The incus may show as a shadow through a thin drum.

9   The chorda tympani   The chorda tympani is the nerve of taste to the anterior $\frac{2}{3}$rds of the tongue (excluding the circumvallate papillae), and is also secretomotor nerve to the submandibular and sublingual salivary glands. The chorda tympani usually lies behind the pars flaccida and is not visible, but if the nerve is more inferior it shows through the drum.

If examination of the drum and meatus is normal in a patient complaining of earache, the pain is referred. *Referred otalgia* may be from nearby structures such as the temporo-mandibular joint, neck muscles or cervical spine; it may be from the teeth, tongue, tonsils or larynx. The Vth, IXth and Xth cranial nerves which supply these sites have their respective tympanic and auricular branches supplying the ear. Earache also frequently precedes a Bell's palsy.

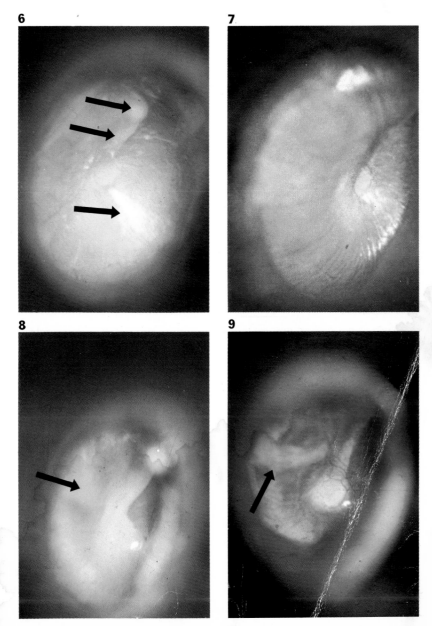

DEAFNESS

10 Conductive and perceptive deafness A patient with deafness has either a conductive or a perceptive loss. The perceptive deafness (also called sensori-neural deafness) is either due to a cochlear or retrocochlear lesion. It is important to diagnose the type of deafness.

The diagnosis is usually clear with simple tests, and most deafnesses fall into a well-defined conductive or perceptive type. ('Mixed' deafness may occur but this diagnosis is usually non-contributory and the term is better avoided).

Lesions to the left of the thick line cause conductive deafness and are frequently curable. Deafness to the right of the thick line is due to a sensori-neural lesion and is usually not amenable to treatment.

Types of Deafness

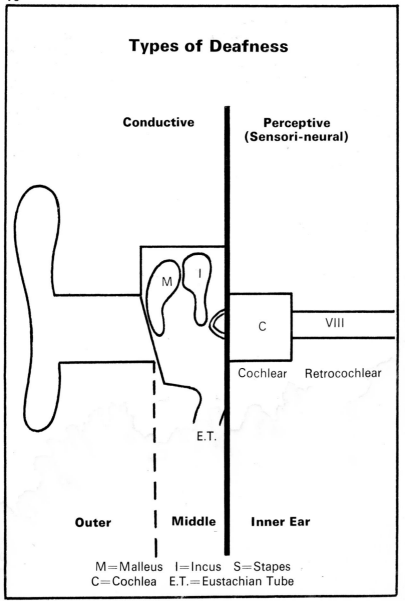

Conductive

**Perceptive
(Sensori-neural)**

M

I

C

VIII

Cochlear   Retrocochlear

E.T.

Outer | **Middle** | **Inner Ear**

M=Malleus   I=Incus   S=Stapes
C=Cochlea   E.T.=Eustachian Tube

TESTS OF DEAFNESS

11 & 12   The Rinne Test   The tuning fork tests are essential preliminary tests for the diagnosis of deafness. The *Rinne* and *Weber* tests enable the diagnosis of conductive or perceptive deafness to be made. If the tuning fork is heard louder on the mastoid process than in front of the ear, the Rinne is *negative* and the deafness is conductive. If the tuning fork is heard better in front of the ear the Rinne is *positive* and the hearing is either normal or there is a perceptive deafness.

13   The Weber test   The tuning fork when held in the midline on the forehead is heard in the ear with the conductive deafness. This test is very sensitive and if the meatus is occluded with the finger, the tuning fork is heard in that ear. A conductive loss of as little as five decibels will result in the Weber being referred to that ear.

14   The occlusion test (Bing) is also helpful. The tuning fork is held on the mastoid process and the tragus lightly pushed to occlude the meatus. The tuning fork is heard louder. In conductive deafness, even of a slight degree, there is no change when the meatus is occluded. The Rinne test does not become negative until there is quite a marked degree of conductive loss (about a 20 decibel air-bone gap). It is therefore possible to have a slight conductive deafness with a positive Rinne. The more sensitive occlusion test will help in the diagnosis.

11

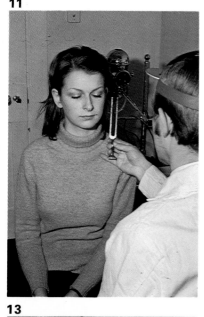

12

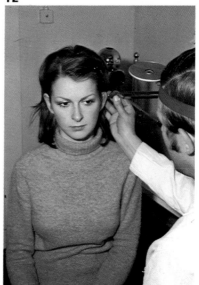

13

14

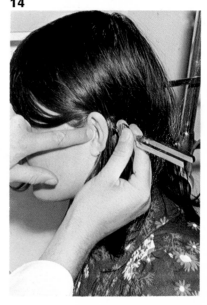

Total deafness in one ear is frequently wrongly diagnosed as a conductive deafness. The Rinne is negative, because the tuning fork, although not heard in front of the ear, when placed on the mastoid process of the deaf ear, is heard by the better ear, the sound being transmitted by the bone (False negative Rinne). The Weber should give the clue that the Rinne is false, for it will not lateralise to the deaf ear.

15   Barany box   This is used to confirm the diagnosis of total deafness. It is placed on the good ear and produces a noise totally masking this ear. The patient will be unable to repeat words clearly spoken into the deaf ear.

Total deafness in one ear may be congenital or result from a skull fracture. Meningitis is also a cause, but *mumps* is probably the commonest cause of this type of deafness. An acoustic neuroma may present with a unilateral perceptive loss, frequently total. If this type of deafness is associated with a canal paresis on the caloric test, and an enlarged internal auditory meatus on x-ray, an acoustic tumour is probable. These are basic preliminary tests in the diagnosis of early acoustic neuromas.

16   Polytomogram x-ray of the internal auditory meatus   This is now one of the most helpful investigations in the diagnosis of an early acoustic tumour.

15

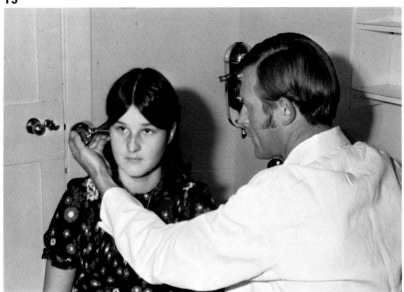

16

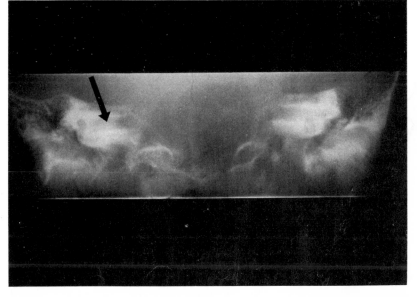

INVESTIGATION OF DEAFNESS

17 Audiometry *A pure tone audiogram* is the standard test of hearing level. The readings are recorded on a chart with intensity (0–100 decibels) and frequency (usually 250–8000 c.p.s.). A normal tracing is between −10dB and +10dB at all frequencies. This test is accurate to about 10 decibels only for there are variables in the patient's responses, and the audiometrician and the machine's accuracy. Hearing is tested in front of the ear (air conduction — recorded in black) and over the mastoid process (bone conduction — in red).

18 Audiograms The one on the left shows a typical perceptive deafness with a high tone loss: a sharp dip at 4000 c.p.s. as on this chart is typical of inner ear damage due to *noise trauma.* A loss of high ' frequencies is commonly seen in senile deafness—*presbycusis.*

The audiogram on the right shows a conductive deafness with the sound heard better on the bone, typical of *otosclerosis*, or *otitis media*.

Audiometry requires skill and training, particularly to test children. An audiogram is obtainable from most children by the age of 3–4. With unilateral deafness, noise is used to mask the better ear, so that this ear does not hear the sound by transmission from the deaf ear and give a false reading. Hearing assessment under the age of 3, or in children who are unable to cooperate with audiometry, requires special skills and techniques. Response of a baby or toddler to meaningful sounds, such as a spoon 'chinked' against a cup, gives an indication of hearing. Cortical evoked response audiometry (CERA) and electrocochleography are two recent tests giving objective hearing levels: the changes in the electroencephalogram recording with auditory stimulus forms the basis of CERA: electrocochleography involves placing fine electrodes through the drum to pick up auditory nerve action potential in response to sound.

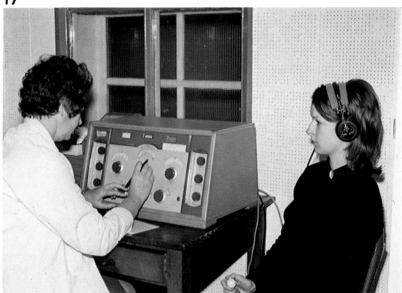

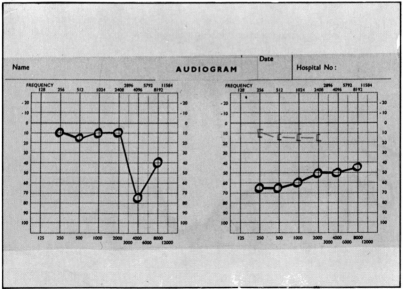

21

19 Bekesy audiometry This gives a more complete and accurate test of hearing than a pure tone audiogram. The response to both interrupted and continuous sound over a wide range of frequencies is recorded. Certain patterns of tracing are associated with types of perceptive deafness, which help in diagnosis. It is possible to distinguish cochlear from retrocochlear deafness and this is an important investigation for acoustic neuroma. This audiogram shows a high tone hearing loss due to presbycusis. With retrocochlear lesions hearing for continuous sound fatigues and the tracing therefore separates from that of interrupted sound.

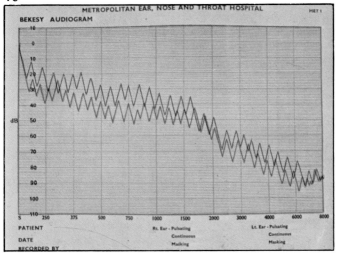

20 & 21   Impedance audiometry   This involves several measurements giving a wide range of information about the middle and inner ear. A metal probe containing three small patent tubes is fitted into the meatus with a soft eartip to make an airtight seal. One tube delivers the tone to the ear, one is attached to a microphone to monitor the sound pressure level within the ear canal, and the third is attached to a manometer to vary the air pressure in the ear. The measurements are particularly helpful in the differential diagnosis of conductive deafness, and also give information about the middle ear pressure and Eustachian tube function, and the level of a lower motor neurone facial nerve palsy.

20

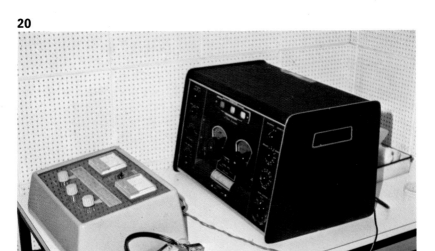

21

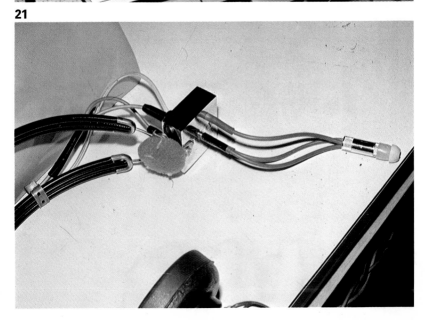

TESTS OF BALANCE

Vertigo is most commonly due to a disorder of the labyrinth. A sensation of unsteadiness may however occur with hypoglycaemia, orthostatic hypotension, hyperventilation and cerebral ischaemia; tumours or multiple sclerosis involving the vestibular system also cause imbalance.

22 Observation for nystagmus is one of the clinical tests for abnormalities of balance. Nystagmus due to a labyrinth disorder is characterised by a slow and quick phase of eye movement: the eye moves slowly away from the side of the involved labyrinth, and flicks rapidly back to that side; the nystagmus is said to be in the direction of the quick phase. The eye movement in nystagmus is fine, and observation of this sign is facilitated if the patient is fitted with glasses with magnifying lenses — Frenzel glasses.

23 The Romberg test is another basic test of balance. This test, in which the patient is asked to stand still with feet together and eyes closed, is made more sensitive by asking the patient to mark time.

24 Tests to demonstrate abnormalities of gait   One of these is heel-toe walking along a straight line : a person with normal balance is stable without looking down at the feet.

Abnormalities in these preliminary clinical tests of balance will indicate the need for further investigation.

22

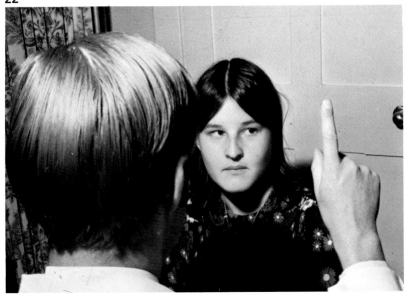

23

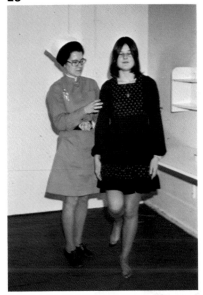

24

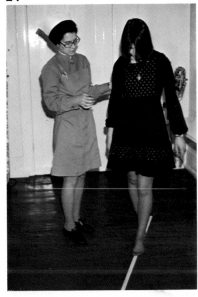

27

Vertigo due to a labyrinth disorder may occur with or without deafness.

25 Positional vertigo *Benign paroxysmal positional vertigo* is a sudden and severe rotary vertigo occurring on lying down in bed, or on looking upwards, when the head is placed backwards and to one side. There is no deafness, and it may follow a head injury. Although common, it is frequently not recognised and unnecessary neurological investigations may be carried out.

The positional history is typical, and the diagnosis is confirmed by a positive positional test: when the head is placed backwards and to one side, nystagmus with vertigo occurs after a short latent period. The nystagmus fatigues within several seconds but recurs temporarily when the patient sits up.

This is a self-limiting condition and simply avoiding the position that triggers off the attack may suffice as treatment. Positional vertigo may also occur with space occupying lesions involving the cerebellum and cerebello-pontine angle. Nystagmus may be induced with the positional test, but there is no latent period and the nystagmus does not fatigue.

26 Vertebro-basilar ischaemia Vertigo with head movement, or transient sudden loss of consciousness ('drop' attacks), occur with temporary interruption of the blood supply to the labyrinth or cerebral cortex. This condition is seen in the older age group with cervical osteoarthritis, and with evidence of hypertension and atherosclerosis. Movement of the irregular cervical spine temporarily occludes the tortuous atherosclerotic vertebral vessels which lead to the basilar and internal auditory arteries.

This *vertebral angiogram* shows the kinking of the vertebral artery.

(*Carotid angiogram by kind permission of Dr Leon Morris, Consultant Radiologist, The London Hospital*)

25

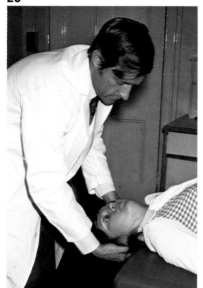

26

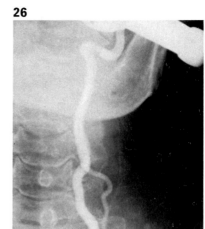

27   The caloric test   Irrigation of the external meatus with water 7° above and later 7° below body temperature sets up convection currents of the endolymph in the semicircular canals. This causes nystagmus and the duration of the nystagmus gives an index of the activity of the labyrinth. The nystagmus can be directly observed or recorded electrically (*electronystagmography*). This test is particularly valuable in the diagnosis of Meniere's disease and acoustic neuroma. A reduced or absent nystagmus is found. (Canal paresis).

28   Meniere's disease   *Sudden severe rotary vertigo* often with nausea and vomiting, a *tinnitus* increasing prior to the vertigo, and a perceptive *deafness* (cochlear type) form the triad of symptoms characteristic of *Meniere's disease.* In this curious condition there is an increase in the endolymph volume, but the cause is unknown. The disease has a reputation for being serious which is not justified. Although the vertigo may occasionally be severe and incapacitating, the symptoms are frequently mild, usually self-limiting and not progressive : it is never fatal, and commonly responds to medical treatment with labyrinthine sedatives, e.g. prochlorperazine ('Stemetil'). Oral histamine-like drugs which aim to increase the blood flow to the inner ear (e.g. 'Serc') promise to be another effective medical treatment. Destruction of the labyrinth and other surgery is rarely needed.

The tinnitus, which is commonly associated with perceptive deafness, is usually not pulsatile. An intermittent or persistent high-pitched ringing noise is heard by the patient: it is difficult to treat, although reassurance (patients frequently associate tinnitus with serious intracranial disease) and the use of tranquillisers is effective, helping the patient to accept tinnitus. Tinnitus may cause serious psychiatric disturbance —particularly with total deafness: the patient may become sufficiently depressed and disturbed to be suicidal. Section of the auditory nerve in the internal auditory meatus may be necessary, although even this radical surgery is not always curative.

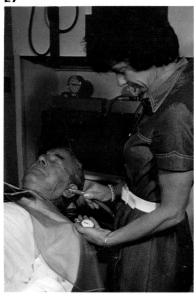

28

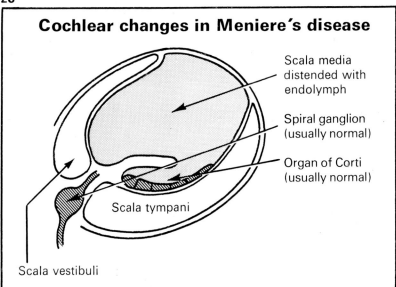

Cochlear changes in Meniere's disease

Scala media distended with endolymph

Spiral ganglion (usually normal)

Organ of Corti (usually normal)

Scala tympani

Scala vestibuli

EXAMINATION OF THE NOSE

29 Examining a child   Instruments are best avoided in children : a good view of the nose anteriorly can be obtained simply by pressing on the tip of the nose. In this case a clear view is obtained of a pedunculated papilloma.

30 A nasal speculum   is needed to see more posteriorly. A simple technique must be learnt to handle this instrument correctly; there are several different types of nasal speculum used throughout the world.

31 The post-nasal space is not easy to examine, particularly in children. With a patient who gags easily, or whose soft palate is close to the posterior wall of the oropharynx, a view may be impossible.

29

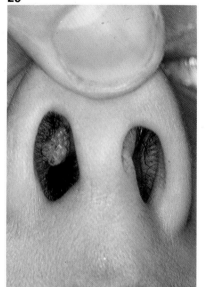

30

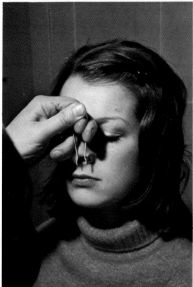

31

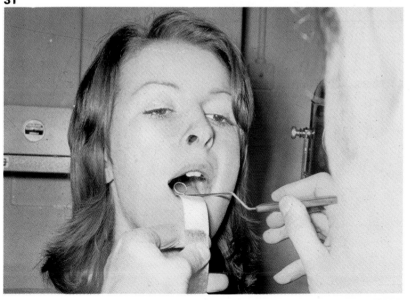

SINUS X-RAYS AND TRANSILLUMINATION

32   X-ray showing maxillary sinus   The sinus most commonly involved in disease is the maxillary sinus. An x-ray will show opacity suggesting infection or polyposis, or opacity with bone destruction suggestive of a neoplasm. The polypoid swelling (shown here in the floor of the left antrum), or thickening of the antral mucosa are frequent chance findings, and in the absence of symptoms or other signs are probably not significant. A straight anterio-posterior x-ray shows the ethmoid and frontal sinuses, and a lateral and base of skull view shows the sphenoid sinus.

33   Transillumination   A bright light held inside the mouth in a dark room is an investigation seldom used now that sinus x-rays are readily available. A dull antrum is however an additional sign in the diagnosis of maxillary sinus disease. Transillumination is useful to assess whether a sinusitis is settling. Dental cysts involving the antrum transilluminate brightly.

32

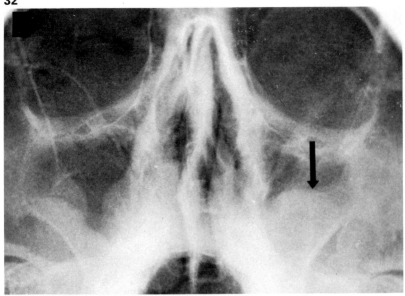

33

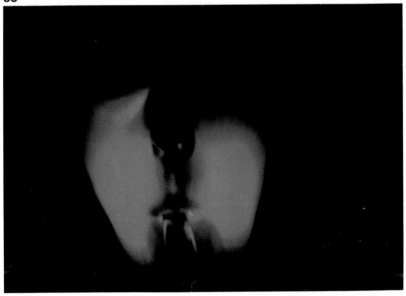

EXAMINING THE PHARYNX AND LARYNX

34   Examination of the pharynx   A tongue depressor is necessary to obtain a clear view of the tonsillar region.

35   Examination of the larynx using the laryngeal mirror (indirect laryngoscopy)   A good view of the larynx is easily obtained with most patients: the valleculae, pyriform fossae, arytenoids, ventricular bands and cords should all be clearly seen. It requires some inhibition of the gag reflex by the patient, and a local anaesthetic lozenge or spray may be necessary. The tongue is held between the thumb and middle finger and the upper lip retracted with the index finger. This examination is difficult in children not only because they may be uncooperative, but because the infantile epiglottis is curved, unlike the 'flat' adult epiglottis, and occludes a clear view of the larynx. Direct laryngoscopy under anaesthetic is usually necessary, therefore, to diagnose the cause of hoarseness in a child. Fibreoptic instruments for laryngoscopy have recently been developed and are a further useful technique in seeing the larynxes of adults and children, which may be difficult on indirect examination.

34

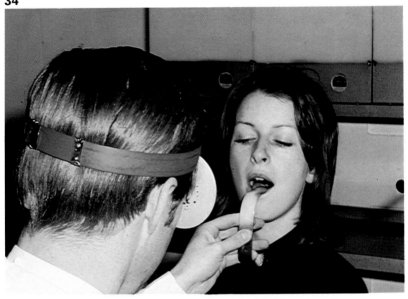

35

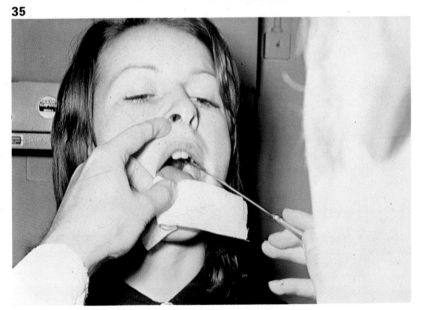

36 **Laryngeal tomogram** This shows the cords (*lower arrow*) and ventricular bands (*upper arrow*), and is used to confirm the site and extent of a lesion. Small lesions on the cord can be detected, and 'hidden sites' in the larynx such as the ventricle and subglottic region are well demonstrated.

37 **Laryngogram** Contrast medium x-rays of the larynx are little used. Although the anatomy is well shown, good pictures are technically difficult to achieve, and require a lot of patience by the subject and radiologist. Good tomograms have tended to displace the laryngogram as an investigation.

36

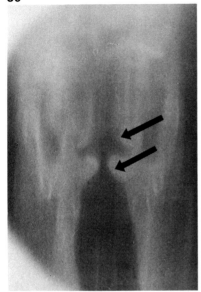

37

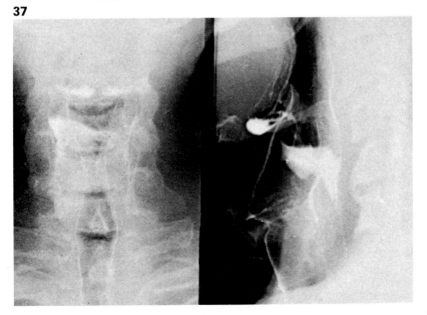

TASTE AND SMELL

38 Solutions used to test taste and smell Four solutions are used to test taste. The solution is placed on one side of the tongue and the patient asked to identify the taste, whether sweet, salt, sour or bitter. This is a relatively crude qualitative test.

Testing for anosmia is with a series of smell solutions for the patient to recognise. Quantitative tests are not in routine clinical use.

Anosmia may be a complication of fracture of the anterior cranial fossa, or it may follow influenza: recovery is uncommon. Temporary anosmia will occur with severe nasal obstruction. Anosmia is invariably linked with a complaint of impaired taste: taste is usually found to be normal on testing and the sensation of smell is an adjunct to the full subtle appreciation of taste.

One is dependent on the integrity of the patient's response to smell and taste tests. It is, therefore, often impossible to be certain in medico-legal cases whether anosmia or ageusia is genuine. With smell, a failure to identify a very strong stimulus such as ammonia suggests malingering, for the Vth and not the Ist cranial nerve is involved.

39 Electrogustometry Electricity has a metallic taste and when a small current in microamps is applied to the tongue, a quantitative reading can be obtained. The normal threshold on the margin of the tongue is between 5 and 30 μa. This more refined test is now widely used in clinical practice and is of value in conditions in which taste may be impaired, such as facial palsy or acoustic neuromas.

38

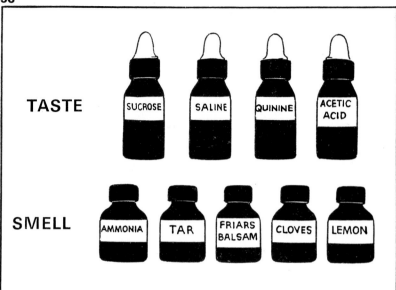

TASTE | SUCROSE | SALINE | QUININE | ACETIC ACID

SMELL | AMMONIA | TAR | FRIARS BALSAM | CLOVES | LEMON

39

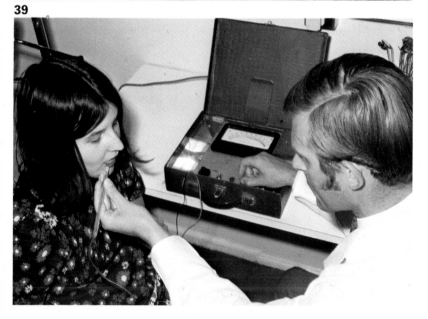

40   The taste buds   These are mainly situated on the tongue and palate, and are centered on the fungiform and circumvallate papillae.

The fungiform papillae (*arrowed*) degenerate with age, and are prominent on a child's tongue. They also atrophy, as seen here, with the loss of the chorda tympani nerve, which may be divided in ear surgery.

41   Circumvallate papillae   These are often prominent on the base of the tongue. A patient may be alarmed when looking at the tongue to notice these normal structures and mistakes them for serious disease. The foliate linguae on the margin of the tongue near the anterior pillar of the fauces may cause similar concern.

The *top arrow* indicates the circumvallate papillae. The *bottom arrow* points to the foliate linguae.

40

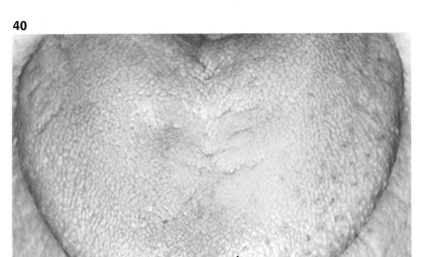

41

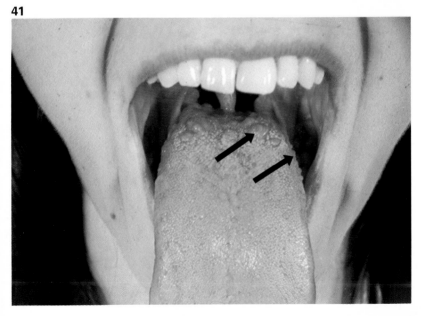

The Ear

THE PINNA

The pinna is formed from the coalescence of six tubercles and *developmental abnormalities* are common.

42   Minor deformities are of little importance. This shows duplication of the lobule.

43   Microtia   Absence of the pinna or gross deformity is often associated with meatal atresia and ossicular abnormalities. Faulty development in the 1st and 2nd branchial arches results in aural deformities which may be associated with hypoplasia of the maxilla and mandible and eye lid deformities (Treacher-Collins syndrome).
   This type of pinna is difficult to treat. Multiple surgical procedures are necessary for reconstruction and a near normal pinna rarely achieved. It may, therefore, be better to advise no treatment or a prosthesis, rather than reconstruction.

44   Darwin's tubercle   A deformity of the pinna of phylogenetic interest. It is homologous to the tip of the mammalian ear and may be sufficiently prominent to justify surgical excision.

42

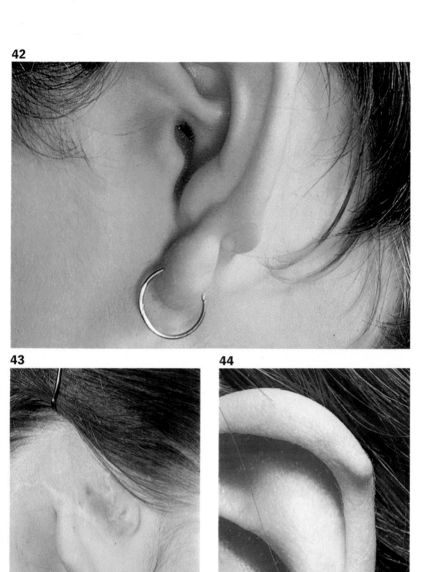

43

44

45 **Hillocks** (or accessory auricles) are common anterior to the tragus and are excised for cosmetic reasons. A small nodule of cartilage is found underlying these hillocks.

46 **Pre-auricular sinuses** which are anterior to the crus of the helix cause more problems. Discharge with recurrent swelling and inflammation may occur. The small opening of the sinus is easily missed on examination, and a furuncle or recurrent furuncles in this site strongly suggest an infected sinus.

Excision when the infection is quiescent is necessary, and this, although minor surgery, is not easy. A long tract often containing cartilage must be dissected out. If the sac is injected with a dye it is better defined. Incomplete excision of the tract leads to further infection and the need for revision surgery.

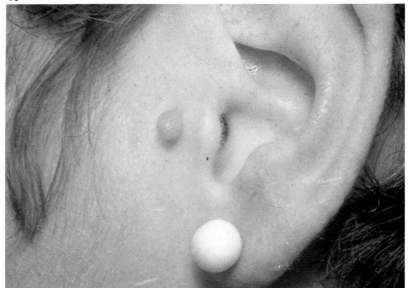

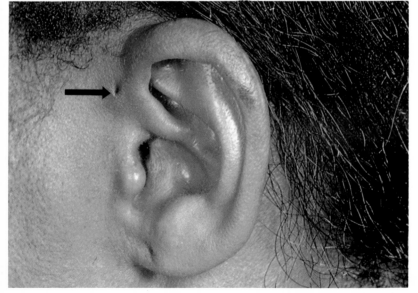

47–50 Prominent Ears The fold of the antihelix is either absent or poorly formed in a prominent ear : parents and child may be offended by the diagnosis of Bat or Lop ears (**47** and **48**).

Surgical correction (**49** and **50**) aims to give a natural looking ear. Modern techniques avoid a 'pinned back' ear with a sharp tender antihelix. Reshaping of the cartilage of the pinna is necessary and recurrence follows simple excision of post-auricular skin.

Prominent ears are probably best corrected between the age of four and six at the beginning of schooling, but there is no additional surgical problem in correcting adult ears.

47

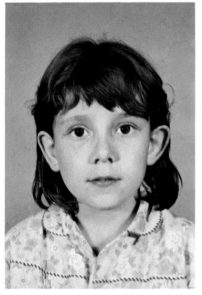

48

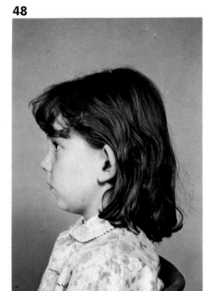

49

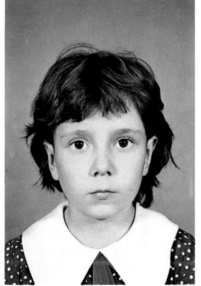

50

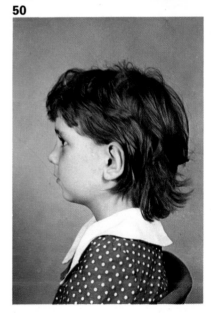

51   Keloid formation is common in Negroes and is difficult to treat. Recurrence follows excision and repeated excision may lead to huge keloid formation.

52   A pre-auricular keloid followed attempts to excise a pre-auricular sinus. Radiotherapy or local triamcinolone injections following excision reduce the incidence of recurrence of the keloid.

53   Nickel sensitivity limits the use of certain ear-rings.

54   Traumatic 'cutting-out' when the ear-ring is pulled by a baby or adult in ill-humour. Infection at the time the sleepers are inserted is another hazard.

51

52

53

54

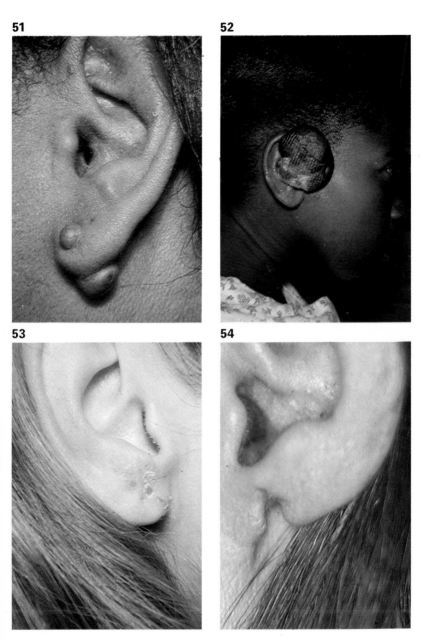

55   Perichondritis   A painful red and swollen pinna, accompanied by fever, following trauma or surgery suggests infection of the cartilage. The organism is frequently Pseudomonas pyocyaneus.

56   Collapse of the pinna cartilage followed perichondritis prior to antibiotics, and perichondritis is still a worrying complication requiring intensive antibiotic treatment. The pinna cartilage may also collapse or alter in shape in *relapsing polychondritis* which is a rare inflammatory condition involving destruction and replacement with fibrous tissue of body cartilage. The larynx too is affected causing hoarseness which may proceed to stridor. The nasal septum may collapse. One or more of the lower limb joints are usually swollen and painful.

57   Haematoma of the pinna may follow trauma. A large haematoma requires incision and a firm dressing to avoid the development of a 'cauliflower ear'.

58   B.I.P. sensitivity   An ear dressing commonly used contains Bismuth, Iodoform and Paraffin (B.I.P.). Sensitivity to iodoform may occur and a red ear with marked *irritation* suggests this complication, (rather than perichondritis which is characterised by *pain*). Early removal of the dressing will prevent a spread of eczema to the pinna, face and neck. A similar skin reaction will occur with a dressing impregnated with an antibiotic or antiseptic to which the patient is allergic.

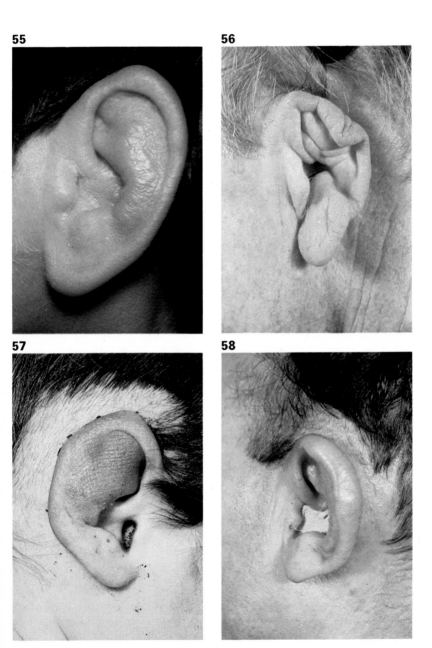

59 & 60   Erysipelas is caused by haemolytic streptococci entering fissures in the skin near the orifice of the ear meatus (fissures such as those in otitis externa). A well-defined raised erythema spreads to involve the face. This condition, serious in pre-antibiotic era, settles rapidly with penicillin.

61 & 62   Herpes zoster   In the head and neck, the herpes zoster virus may affect the *Gasserian ganglion* of the Vth cranial nerve. In **61** the mandibular and maxillary divisions are involved. The vesicular type of skin eruption is confined to the distribution of the nerve. The ophthalmic division of V is most frequently involved, but all three divisions of V are rarely affected at the same time.

The herpes zoster virus also involves the *geniculate ganglion* of the VIIth cranial nerve (Ramsey-Hunt syndrome or geniculate herpes): herpes affects the pinna and pre-auricular region(**62**) and is associated with a facial palsy. In most cases, there is also vertigo and perceptive deafness. There is less likelihood of a full recovery of the facial palsy than in Bell's palsy.

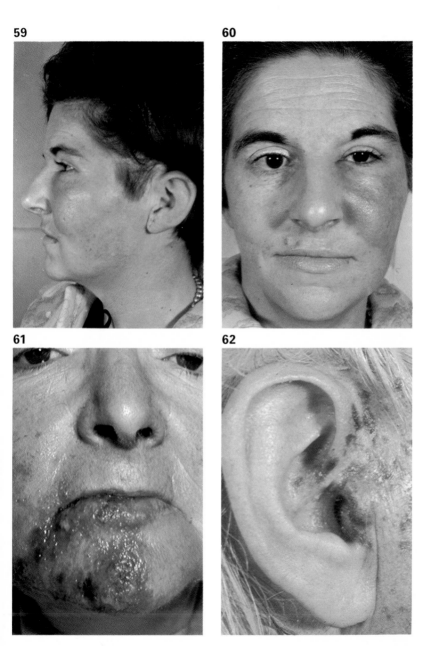

63 Basal cell carcinoma Ulceration is not uncommon on the helix ; a long history suggests a *basal cell carcinoma*. This is treated with wedge resection. An ulcer of short duration suggests a squamous cell carcinoma or more rarely a melanoma, both of which require more extensive surgical resection.

64 Solar keratoses These warty growths affect the skin of the fairhaired exposed to strong sunlight. They may become malignant. The skin of the helix may be affected with several of these keratoses.

65 Inflammatory ulcers These affect the helix and occasionally the antihelix. The lesions on the helix are blessed with a lengthy diagnosis—*chondrodermatitis nodularis helicis chronicis*, which presents as a long standing intermittent ulceration. It is primarily a chronic chondritis with secondary skin infection. A wedge resection of the ulcer and cartilage may be necessary for the ulcer does not heal with ointments.

63

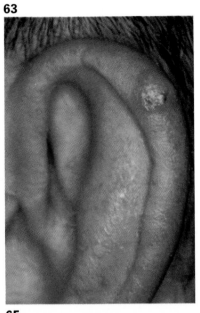

64

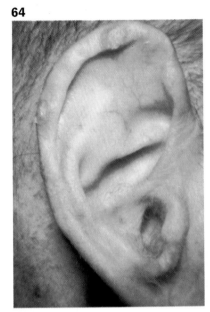

65

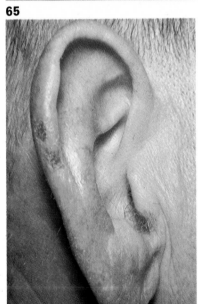

66 Ulcers of the antihelix These are usually traumatic (on a particularly prominent antihelix fold) and are primarily a skin lesion. A basal or squamous cell carcinoma may, however, present on the antihelix.

67 Gouty tophi also occur on the helix.

(Picture by kind permission of Dr A H Davies, Chepstow)

66

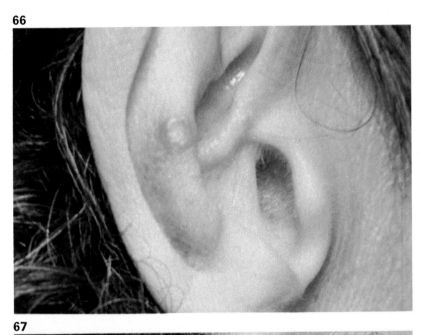

67

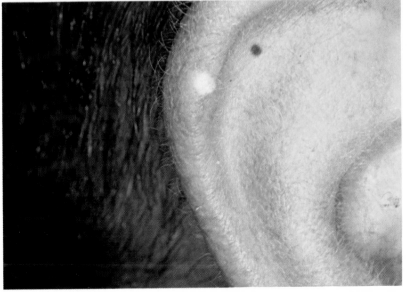

THE EXTERNAL AUDITORY MEATUS

The skin of the external auditory meatus is migratory and does not desquamate.

68–71 **A migrating ink dot** A dot of ink, if placed near the centre of the drum (**68**), is found to lie near the margin of the drum in 3 weeks (**69**) and between 6–12 weeks the dot migrates outwards on the meatal skin (**70, 71**) to emerge in wax at the orifice of the meatus.

Cleaning of the ear canal is therefore unnecessary: those who diligently clean their ears, or those of their children, with cotton buds etc., hinder the migration of skin, and wax tends to accumulate and otitis externa develop. The migration of meatal epithelium is also abnormal in *keratosis obturans:* in this condition desquamated epithelium accumulates and may form a large impacted mass in the meatus causing erosion of the bony canal.

Skin grafts initially used for myringoplasty often failed or led to otitis externa, because skin taken from elsewhere on the body did not take on this migratory role: fascia is now used to graft the ear drum.

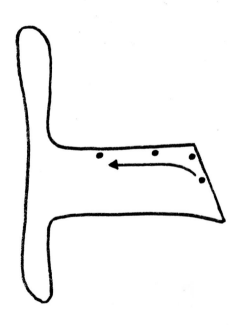

68

69

70

71

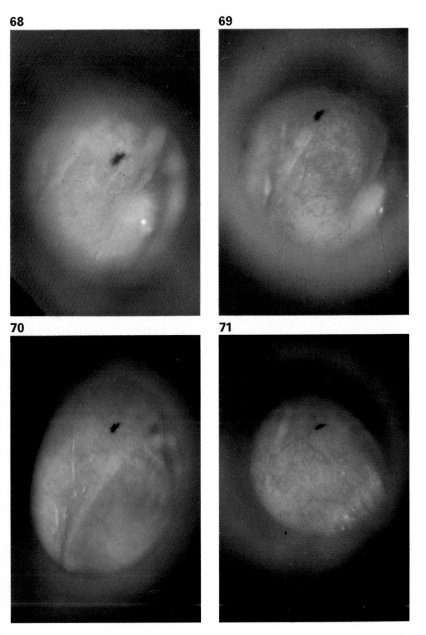

Although wax normally does not accumulate because of meatal skin migration, it may impact and cause a hearing loss.

72 & 73   Syringing is simple and effective treatment. The pinna is pulled outwards and backwards to straighten the meatus and water at body temperature is irrigated along the posterior wall of the ear. The water finds a passage past the wax, rebounds off the drum and pushes the wax outwards. Hard wax may require the use of drops before syringing.

Syringing is not painful and pain means an error in technique, or that there is an otitis externa or a perforation. If there is a perforation, an ear should not be syringed: pain with vertigo may occur with subsequent otitis media and otorrhoea; a past history of discharge suggests a perforation. Coughing (from the vagal reflex—the auricular branch of the vagus supplies the drum) or syncope may complicate syringing. Vertigo with nystagmus will occur if the water is too hot or too cold.

74   Foreign body in the ear   *The main danger of a foreign body in the ear lies in its careless removal.* Syringing is very effective and safe for small metallic foreign bodies. Vegetable foreign bodies, such as peas, swell with water and are better not syringed. Insects not uncommonly become impacted in the meatus, particularly in the tropics. Maggots cause a painful ear and their removal is difficult: insufflation of pulv. calomel is usually effective treatment. Previous attempts to remove a piece of plastic wedged in this child's meatus (**74**) have led to bleeding in the meatus: the drum against which the foreign body impinges can be seen deep to the plastic. One must *not* persevere in attempts to remove an aural foreign body, particularly in a child: a perforation is easily caused. If immediate removal with a hook or syringe is not effective, the patient must be admitted for removal under general anaesthetic with the help of the microscope. It is often dangerous to use forceps to remove an aural foreign body: the object easily slips from the jaws of the forceps to go deeper into the meatus.

72

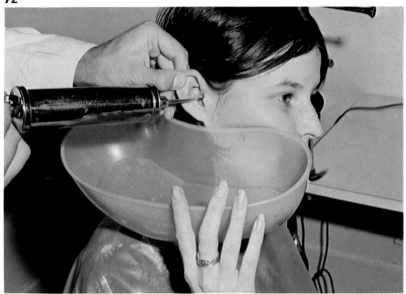

73

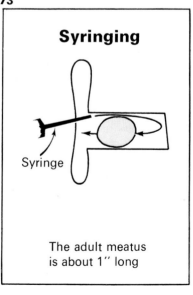

Syringing

Syringe

The adult meatus
is about 1″ long

74

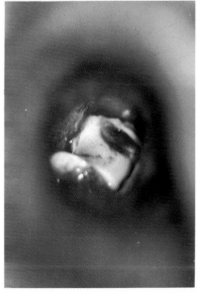

75   Otitis externa   Eczema of the meatus and pinna (seen here) may be associated with eczema elsewhere, particularly in the scalp, or it may be an isolated condition affecting only one ear. *Itching* is the main symptom, with scanty discharge. The eczematous type of otitis externa usually settles with cleaning of the meatus, followed by the use of a topical corticosteroid and antibiotic, but recurrence is not uncommon. The patient should avoid over-diligent cleaning of the meatus, scratching the ear, and should prevent water entering the meatus during washing or swimming: these are some of the factors predisposing to recurrence.

76   Eardrop sensitivity   Sensitivity to ear drops may worsen an otitis externa. Chloramphenicol drops were responsible for this condition. Neomycin less commonly causes a similar reaction. Patients should be advised to discontinue ear drops that cause an increase in irritation or are painful.

77   A furuncle in the meatus is the other common type of otitis externa. It is characterised by *pain*: pain on movement of the pinna or on inserting the auriscope is diagnostic of a furuncle. Diabetes mellitus must be excluded with recurrent furuncles.

78   Furunculosis   This is a generalised infection of the meatal skin. Pain is severe and the canal is narrowed or occluded so that examination with the auriscope is extremely painful and no view of the deep meatus is possible. A swab of the pus should be taken and treatment is with systemic antibiotics and a meatal dressing (e.g. glycerine and ichthyol, or a corticosteroid cream with an antibiotic). The organism may be transferred by the patient's finger from the nasal vestibules and a nasal swab is a relevant investigation, particularly with recurrent furuncles. The lymph nodes adjacent to the pinna are enlarged with a furuncle or furunculosis and a tender mastoid node may mimic a cortical mastoid abscess.

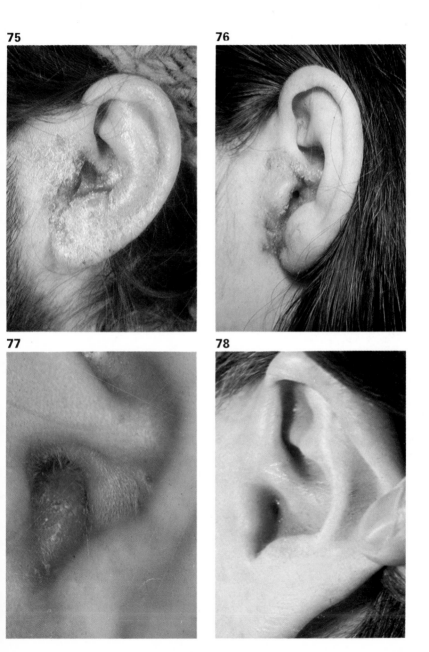

79 & 80 Otitis externa is initially treated with cleaning of the meatus and the instillation of the appropriate antibiotic and corticosteroid drops. If the condition persists and irritation and pain are marked, a **fungal otitis externa** should be suspected. In persistent infection, the meatus contains a cocktail of drops, pus and desquamated skin. In fungal infections, as shown here, the dark spores and white mycelium can be seen. Thorough cleaning of the meatus precedes treatment with a topical antifungal agent.

The meatal skin infection is introduced from outside—usually from the patient's finger, or from water, particularly after swimming. The infection, however, may be from the middle ear if there is a perforation, and discharge from chronic otitis media may be the cause of a persistent otitis externa (**79**).

81 Bullous otitis externa (bullous myringitis) This unusual otitis externa frequently follows influenza or an upper respiratory tract infection. A complaint of earache followed by *bleeding*, followed by relief of pain is diagnostic of this condition. Examination shows haemorrhagic blebs on the drum and meatus, similar to the vesicular eruption of herpes. If there is pyrexia with a conductive deafness, the otitis externa is associated with an otitis media and systemic antibiotics are necessary. In the absence of pyrexia and hearing loss this condition settles spontaneously without treatment.

82 Otitis externa with herpes zoster Otitis externa occurs with herpes zoster involving either the Gasserian or geniculate ganglion, and the vesicles may be haemorrhagic.

Carcinomas and melanomas in the skin of the external auditory meatus are rare but any persistent granulation should be biopsied. A rare but extremely serious type of otitis externa occurs in elderly diabetics, and is characterised by granulation tissue in the meatus, infected with Pseudomonas pyocyaneus. This condition is called 'malignant otitis externa' and, although inflammatory rather than neoplastic, this is an apposite label, for the granulation tissue tends to erode via the middle ear and labyrinth to the brain, or to the great vessels of the neck. This condition has a high mortality from intracranial complication or haemorrhage, despite intensive antibiotic therapy and surgery to remove the infected granulation tissue.

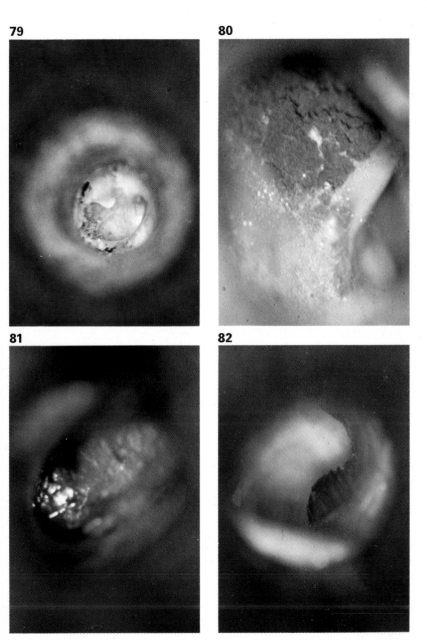

83 Osteomas White bony hard swellings in the deep meatus are a common finding during a routine examination. They usually remain small and are symptom free. They tend to be symmetrical in both ears. Swimmers are susceptible to these lesions which are sometimes called 'swimmer's osteomas'. There is experimental evidence to show that irrigation of the bony meatus with cold water produces a periostitis that leads to osteoma formation. Although the term osteoma is widely used for this condition, it is not histologically a neoplasm and the term exostosis is probably more correct.

84 Large osteomas may narrow the meatus to a chink so that wax accumulates and is difficult to syringe. Otitis externa is also a complication. These osteomas may, therefore, require surgical removal with a microdrill. They should not be removed with a gouge, for a fracture and bleeding within the remaining osteoma is a probable complication, causing damage to the facial nerve, and resulting in facial palsy. It is extremely rare for osteomas to occlude the meatus completely, and in almost all cases no treatment is required.

83

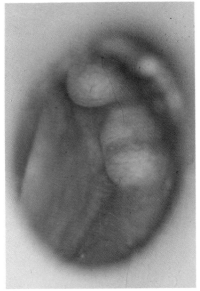

84

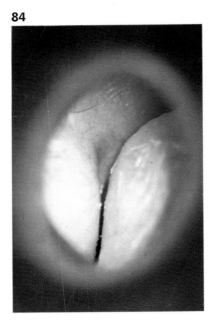

THE TYMPANIC MEMBRANE AND MIDDLE EAR

85, 86 & 87 'Chalk' patches   White areas of *tympanosclerosis* are common findings on examination of the drum. They are of little significance in themselves and the hearing is often normal. A past history of otorrhoea in childhood is usual, but chalk patches do occur with no apparent past otitis media.

Extensive tympanosclerosis with a rigid drum is a sequel of past otitis media and the ossicles too may be fixed or not in continuity. The chorda tympani is visible through the tympanic membrane in **85**.

88   Scarring of the drum   Scarring of the drum with retraction onto the promontory, incus and round window is also evidence of past otitis media. It is sometimes difficult to be sure whether this type of drum is intact: a thin layer of epithelium indrawn onto the middle ear structures may seal the middle ear, and examination with a Siegle's speculum or the operating microscope may be necessary to be certain of an intact drum.

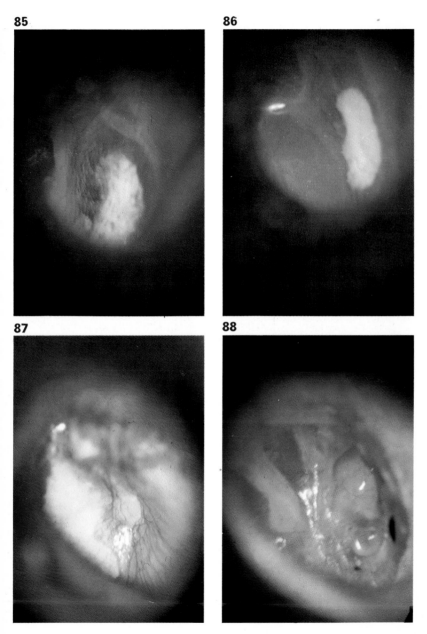

Perforations of the tympanic membrane may be caused by trauma or infection (otitis media).

89, 90 & 91 Traumatic perforation   A blow on the ear with the hand is a common cause of a traumatic perforation. The traumatic perforation has an irregular margin and there is fresh blood or blood clot on the drum (**90**). The defect is frequently slit-shaped (**91**). Pain and transient vertigo at the time of injury are followed by a tinnitus and hearing loss.

92 Healing perforation   Almost all traumatic perforations heal spontaneously within two months, a thin membrane growing across the defect.

Traumatic perforations are usually central but if the perforation extends to the annulus healing may not occur. Care to avoid water entering the middle ear and avoidance of inflating the middle ear with the Valsalva manoeuvre are the only precautions the patient need take. A middle ear infection with discharge is the commonest complication which usually settles with a course of topical and systemic antibiotics.

Blast injuries, barotrauma, foreign bodies or their careless removal, and even over-enthusiastic kissing of the ear may also cause traumatic perforations.

89

90

91

92

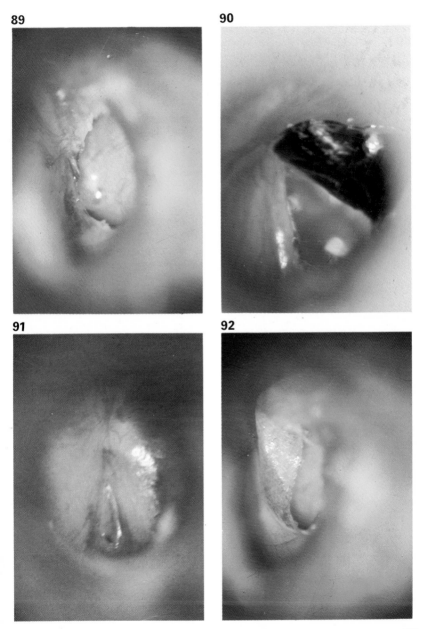

93 Central perforation Acute otitis media with pus under pressure in the middle ear may rupture the drum and although healing usually occurs, a permanent perforation can result. These perforations are usually central. A small perforation may be symptom free but episodes of otorrhoea with head colds and after swimming are common, and there is a conductive deafness.

The otorrhoea tends to be profuse and muco-purulent: it may be intermittent or persistent. This type of central perforation when dry is successfully closed with a fascial graft (myringoplasty). Other complications with central perforations are rare and it is described as a *'safe'* perforation. Myringoplasty in children is usually avoided. The frequency of upper respiratory tract infection, and the relative inefficiency of the child's eustachian tube predisposes to otitis media and break-down of the graft. In children, furthermore, spontaneous closure of central perforations is common. There are occasions, however, when myringoplasty is indicated: with bilateral perforations associated with a significant hearing loss, myringoplasty may be required to avoid the use of a hearing aid. A child, in addition, who has recurrent episodes of otorrhoea which may be related to swimming, may require surgery.

94 Marginal perforation A perforation may reach the annulus posteriorly and is called marginal. The middle ear structures are frequently seen through the perforation. The well-defined margin of the round window is particularly obvious and the promontory, incudo-stapedial joint and stapedius are also apparent.

93

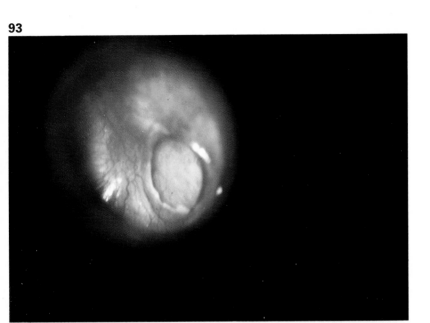

94

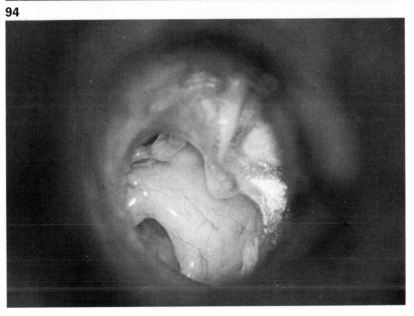

95   Squamous epithelium on the incus   The marginal perforation may enable squamous epithelium to migrate into the middle ear. In this ear, white squamous epithelium has formed on the incus. Marginal perforations, therefore, are described as *'unsafe'* as there is a risk of cholesteatoma. Perforations of the pars flaccida (attic perforations) are invariably associated with cholesteatoma formation.

96   Attic perforation   Debris adherent to the pars flaccida of the drum suggests an underlying attic perforation.

97   Cholesteatoma   The debris, when removed, exposes a white mass of epithelium characteristic of a cholesteatoma. Cholesteatoma is *not* a neoplasm; it is simply squamous epithelium in the middle ear. If ignored, it increases in size, becomes infected and is associated with a scanty fetid otorrhoea. It may erode bone leading to serious complica-cations: extension to involve the dura with intracranial infection may occur, and the facial nerve and labyrinth too may be eroded. The extent of the cholesteatoma determines the danger: a small attic pocket of epithelium is relatively harmless and can be removed with suction; an extensive mass of epithelium is dangerous and needs exploration and removal via a mastoidectomy approach. A chronic discharging ear is not painful, and persistent *pain* and headache, or severe vertigo, strongly suggest an intracranial complication or labyrinthitis.

95

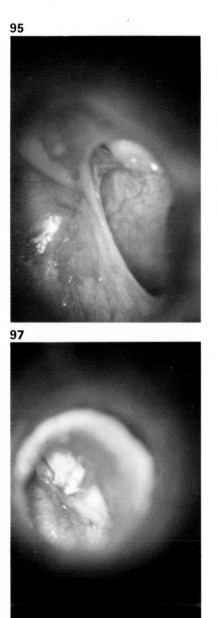

96

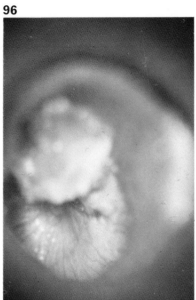

97

98   Cholesteatoma erodes the bony wall of the deep meatus so that a pocket containing white debris forms in the postero-superior aspect of the drum.

The complete aetiology of cholesteatoma is not understood. Migration of epithelium into the middle ear via an attic or posterior marginal perforation certainly accounts for most cholesteatomas. Cholesteatoma may, however, occur behind an intact drum, and may form with central perforations. Eustachian tube dysfunction with a negative pressure in the middle ear, if long-standing, leads to a chronic middle ear effusion (chronic secretory otitis media) and a retracted drum. The pars flaccida retracts and may give the opportunity for a pocket of cholesteatoma to develop. In this picture of cholesteatoma, the remainder of the drum is a golden colour and fluid is present in the middle ear. The secretory otitis media may have been responsible for this cholesteatoma formation.

99 A cholesteatoma removed at mastoidectomy presents the typical well defined mass of white epithelium. The bone erosion that this mass causes shows on mastoid x-ray and particularly well on polytomograms.

98

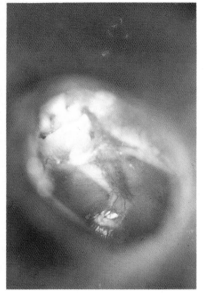

99

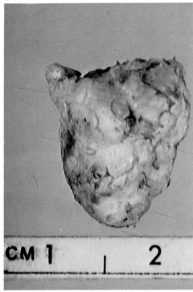

100   Aural granulation   In the same way that epithelium may migrate through a perforation into the middle ear, mucous membrane may extrude outwards into the meatus. Middle ear mucous membrane extruding through a perforation becomes infected and presents with a discharging ear. An aural granulation is seen in the deep meatus. Granulation may also form on the drum at the margin of the perforation, and rarely granulation tissue forms on an intact drum in otitis externa (granular myringitis).

101   Pedunculated polyp   If the growth of granulation tissue is exuberant, a pedunculated *polyp* develops, which may present at the orifice of the meatus. Granulations and polyps commonly arise from the tympanic annulus posteriorly, but the mucous membrane of the promontory, Eustachian tube orifice, and antrum and aditus may also be the site of origin.

Careful and thorough removal of polyps and granulation tissue to their site of origin is necessary. If the polyp is associated with cholesteatoma, removal by mastoid approach is required.

100

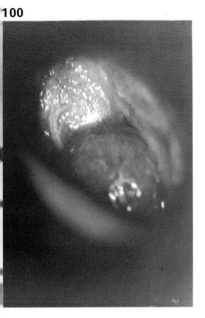

101

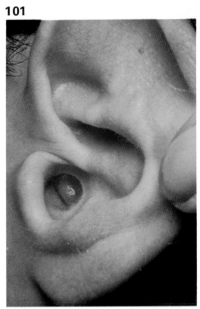

Mastoidectomy   In the past mastoidectomy was needed for acute mastoiditis complicating acute otitis media; this was extremely common in the pre-antibiotic era and required exenteration of the mastoid air cells (cortical mastoidectomy). The operation is now rarely performed in countries where antibiotics are available.

102   Enlarged meatus after mastoidectomy   A more extensive type of mastoidectomy is, however, still necessary for cholesteatoma which has extended beyond the middle ear. This operation alters the anatomy of the ear. Examination after operation will show an enlarged meatus. At operation the meatus is enlarged with a meatoplasty to allow access to the mastoid cavity, so that wax can be removed with a Jobson-Horne probe or with suction. This is usually necessary once or twice a year for the skin of the mastoid cavity does not migrate satisfactorily and wax accumulates. Syringing of a mastoid cavity is avoided, for irrigation of water over the horizontal semicircular canal in the mastoid cavity may cause vertigo, and unless the cavity is dried carefully, infection and discharge occur.

103   Auriscope view   With the auriscope a ridge (which contains the facial nerve) can be seen separating the drum anteriorly from the epithelialised cavity posteriorly. Failure of the mastoid cavity to epithelialise results in an infected cavity with discharge.

Top arrow points to mastoid cavity; *second arrow* indicates the facial ridge with the bone overlying the descending portion of the facial nerve; *third arrow* shows the tympanic membrane.

Recent surgical techniques aim to remove cholesteatoma without exteriorising the mastoid cavity, so that relatively normal anatomy is maintained post-operatively, and hearing is maintained or improved (*intact canal wall tympanoplasty*), although this operation is not suitable for every case.

(*Picture by kind permission of Charles Smith, Consultant Surgeon, York*)

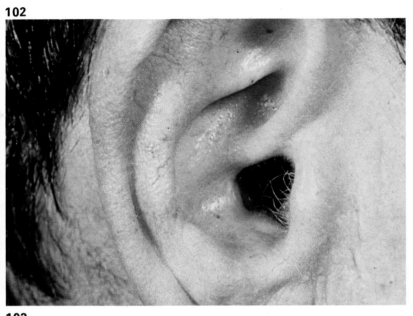

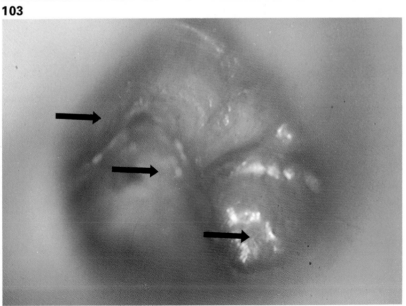

Secretory otitis media   A sterile middle ear exudate is a common cause of conductive deafness. It may occur when either a head cold or barotrauma interfere with Eustachian tube function, and it often follows acute otitis media. A post-nasal space neoplasm may also cause Eustachian tube obstruction and is to be excluded in any adult with a persistent secretory otitis media.

In children secretory otitis media is very common when adenoid tissue interferes with the Eustachian tube. The middle-ear fluid tends to be tenacious ('glue ear'), unlike the thin straw-coloured exudate of adults.

The appearance of the drum is altered and the mobility reduced.

104   Secretory otitis media with minimal drum change   The drum may look only slightly different with a brown colour and some hyperaemia.

105   Secretory otitis media with marked drum change   The change is frequently gross, making the diagnosis obvious, with a golden colour, a retracted membrane and a prominent malleus.

106   A fluid level and bubbles may be seen with secretory otitis media.

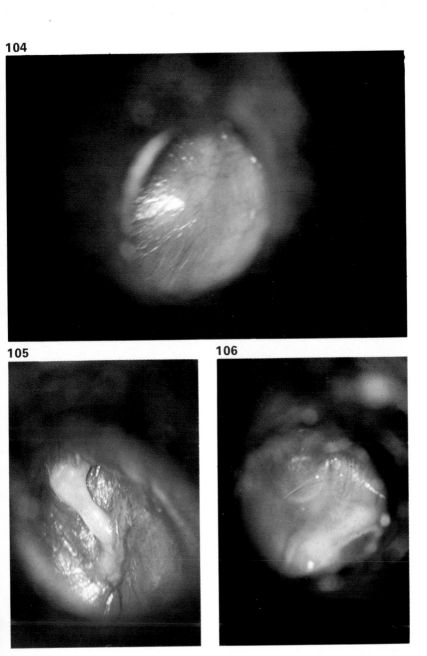

104

105

106

107   A vesicle on the drum also occurs in children's glue ear.

The full aetiology of the Eustachian tube dysfunction causing secretory otitis media is at present unknown. Opinions therefore differ on the treatment, particularly that of children's 'glue ears'. Adenoid tissue in the region of the Eustachian tube orifice predisposes to 'glue ears', and adenoid removal is frequently necessary surgery.

'Glue ears' are common between the ages of 3–6, and rarely persist after 11. The hearing loss is often slight and varies with colds. The self-limiting nature of the condition calls for conservative treatment, *but 'glue ears' are not to be ignored.* A marked and persistent hearing loss, interfering with schooling necessitates surgery. Episodes of transient otalgia are common with 'glue ears', and frequent attacks of acute otitis media may occur: the drum may also become retracted and flaccid with prolonged middle ear fluid. These features may also necessitate the insertion of a gromet to reventilate the middle ear.

108   Blue drum   The middle ear effusion evidently alters in composition, for at some stages in secretory otitis media the drum appears blue in colour—so called 'blue drum'. A similar blue appearance of the drum is seen following head injury with bleeding into the middle ear. At first, a haemotympanum gives a reddish appearance of the drum, but later a blue colour similar to that seen in secretory otitis media develops. Blood in the middle ear usually resolves spontaneously without myringotomy, with a return to normal hearing. Persistent conductive deafness after the drum has returned to normal suggests injury to the ossicular chain, and tympanotomy is indicated.

107

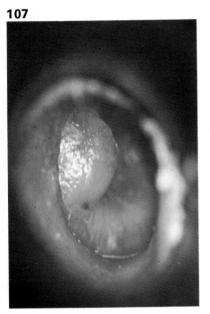

108

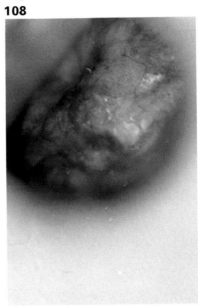

Secretory otitis media may settle spontaneously. Nasal vasoconstrictor drops with an oral decongestant (an antihistamine with a pseudo ephedrine preparation) help recovery, as may insufflation of the Eustachian tube, either by the patient performing the Valsalva manoeuvre, or by Politzerisation or Eustachian catheterisation.

109   Myringotomy   If, however, secretory otitis media with poor hearing persists over six to eight weeks, myringotomy, usually under general anaesthetic, with aspiration of the fluid is often necessary.

110   Gromet   The insertion of a *gromet*, a flanged teflon tube, is frequently needed to avoid a recurrence of middle ear fluid.

111   Gromet insertion   A myringotomy incision in the posterior half of the drum may damage the incudostapedial joint or round window, and a gromet inserted posteriorly may cause incus necrosis from pressure on the long process: an anterior radial myringotomy is a safer incision for gromet insertion (as here). In both adults and children the post-nasal space must be seen to be normal.

112   A gromet in place   The gromet tube ventilates the middle ear and acts instead of the Eustachian tube. Hearing, and the appearance of the drum return to normal.

The gromet usually extrudes spontaneously between four to twelve months and is found in wax in the meatus. If normal Eustachian tube function has not returned and secretory otitis media recurs, the gromet is replaced.

Obstruction of the eustachian tube is a common and frequently diagnosed disorder. *Abnormal patency* of the tube, however is also not uncommon, but the diagnosis is frequently missed. The condition tends to occur in those who have lost weight, those on the Pill, and in pregnancy. The symptoms are of a sensation of blockage in the ear, but with good hearing. The patients may comment that they hear themselves breathe, eat and hear their own voice. Fortunately the symptoms are usually minor and reassurance and explanation suffice as treatment in most cases. Failure to make the diagnosis, however, and treatment of the condition as eustachian tube obstruction is common.

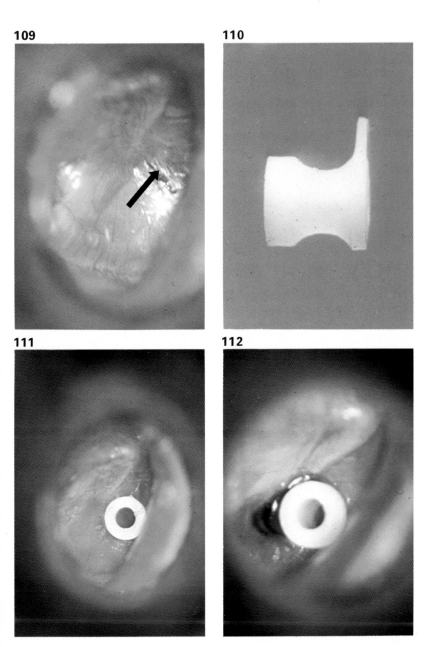

Chronic secretory otitis media   Middle ear fluid if persistent may cause permanent changes in the drum. A secretory otitis media can cause deafness for decades and the diagnosis is frequently overlooked in a longstanding deafness. Impedance audiometry helps in diagnosis.

113   Grossly altered drum   A brown colour, with retraction of a flaccid membrane onto the ossicles and promontory is seen. *Lower arrow* points to indrawn drum; *upper arrow* shows incudo-stapedial joint.

114   Gromet occluded with exudate   Insertion of a gromet in these chronic adult cases may restore hearing but frequently the lumen of the gromet becomes occluded with exudate which may extrude through the tube into the meatus, or a constant otorrhoea occurs. There is no present successful treatment for chronic secretory otitis media failing to respond to insertion of a gromet. A further problem with chronic secretory otitis media is the return of middle ear fluid with deafness when the gromet extrudes. A larger flanged gromet which remains in position longer, and periodic replacement are the only remedies.

113

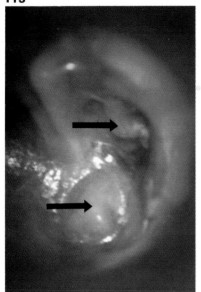

114

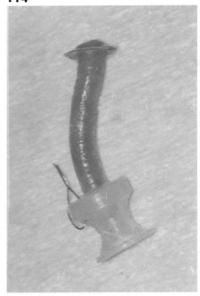

115 Acute otitis media Earache with conductive deafness and fever, accompanying a head cold, characterises acute otitis media. The drum is red and the landmarks are obscured: distension and pulsation may be seen. Otitis media is common in children, probably due to their short, wide Eustachian tube, and the presence of adenoids which may be infected near the orifice. Rupture of the tympanic membrane in acute otitis media is not uncommon and muco-purulent otorrhoea ensues with a pulsatile discharge.

Penicillin is invariably rapidly curative and complications are rare. Acute mastoiditis, previously serious and common, is almost unheard of where antibiotics are available. Myringotomy and cortical mastoidectomy are operations of the past for acute otitis media.

Secretory otitis media after the acute attack is the main complication today.

116 Glomus jugulare tumour may present with a red drum simulating acute otitis media. *There is, however, no pain.* This tumour arises from the chemoreceptor cells near the jugular foramen and the floor of the middle ear. Pulsating tinnitus, a conductive deafness and a red swelling in the hypotympanum (seen here) are diagnostic of this tumour. A large tumour may extrude through the drum and present as a vascular aural polyp.

The histology is similar to the carotid body tumour, with which it may co-exist. If the glomus tumour occupies the middle ear, it can be removed via a tympanotomy or mastoidectomy approach. When the jugular foramen is involved with loss of the IX, X and XIth cranial nerves (often the XIIth from the anterior condular foramen is also affected), the treatment is difficult. A surgical approach has been recently developed via the mastoid and neck, with a neurosurgical exposure if there is an intracranial extension. If the tumour is inaccessible surgically, radiotherapy does slow the growth of an already very slow-growing tumour and has an important place in the management, particularly in the more elderly patient. If ignored, this tumour is fatal, due to intracranial spread.

A red drum may also follow head injury with bleeding into the middle ear. A *haemotympanum* settles without treatment, but a persistent conductive deafness suggests damage to the ossicular chain.

115

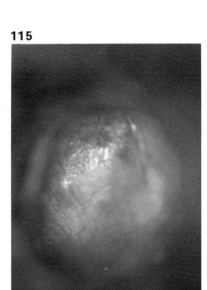

116

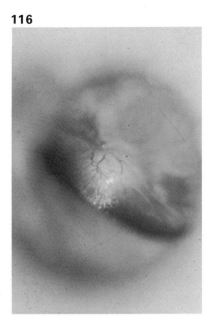

117   Otosclerosis   This is a common cause of bilateral symmetrical conductive deafness in adults. The stapes footplate is ankylosed in the oval window by thick vascular bone : this curious bony lesion is usually an isolated middle ear focus. It may, however, be associated with osteogenesis imperfecta tarda, and *blue sclerae* are occasionally seen with otosclerosis.

Otosclerosis is familial and commoner in women (otosclerotic deafness increases during pregnancy and this may account for the apparent higher incidence in women). Patients frequently notice paracusis, in which they hear more clearly in noisy surroundings, unlike perceptive deafness in which there is difficulty in hearing with background noise. The cause of otosclerosis remains unknown.

118   The stapes   The smallest bone in the body. It is, like the other ossicles, adult size at birth.

117

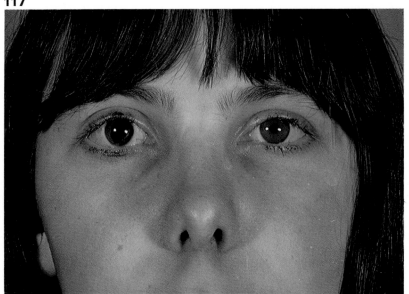

118

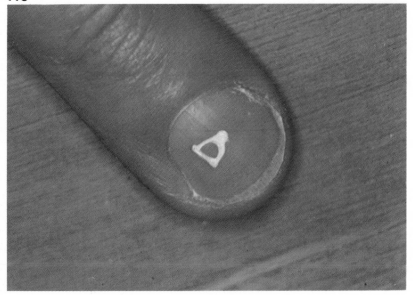

119   Stapedectomy—the prostheses   The operation for deafness due to otosclerosis involves removal of the ankylosed stapes bone and replacement with a mobile prosthesis. There are several types of prosthesis, of which gel-foam wire (*right*), stainless steel (*centre*) or teflon (*left*) are the most commonly used. This very successful operation was devised by John Shea of Memphis, Tennessee, U.S.A., in 1957, and was a great advance in surgery with good hearing achieved in over 90% of cases.

120   An opening is made in the fixed footplate (shown here). The white marks to the right of this opening into the inner ear are the otoliths.

The prosthesis is attached to the long process of the incus, and the distal end of the prosthesis is placed into the inner ear.

121   The stapedectomy operation   The top diagram shows the attachment of the stapes prosthesis to the long process of the incus: the distal end of the prosthesis is placed through the opening made in the ankylosed stapes footplate.

The lower diagram shows the exposure of the middle ear for stapedectomy. The drum is reflected anteriorly, hinging on the long process of the malleus. The stapes superstructure and part of the footplate are removed, and the prosthesis inserted.

119

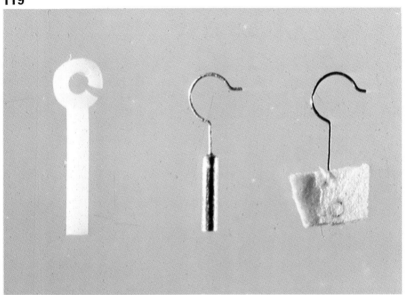

120

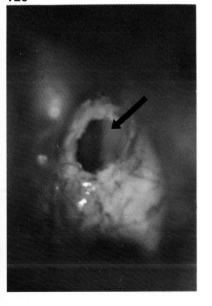

121

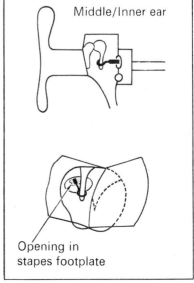

Middle/Inner ear

Opening in
stapes footplate

122 A teflon-wire prosthesis (top arrow) The distal end is entering the inner ear through the hole in the footplate (*bottom arrow*).

123 A gel-foam wire prosthesis The wire loop is closed onto the incus (*top arrow*) and the gel-foam (*second arrow*) becomes replaced in the oval window by a fibrous membrane. The bone covering the facial nerve (*third arrow*) and margin of the round window (*bottom arrow*) are also seen.

122

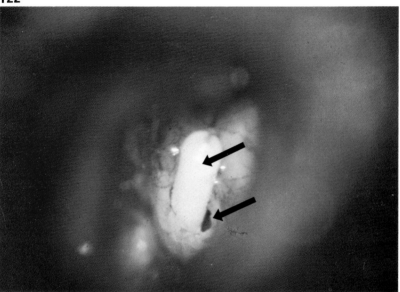

123

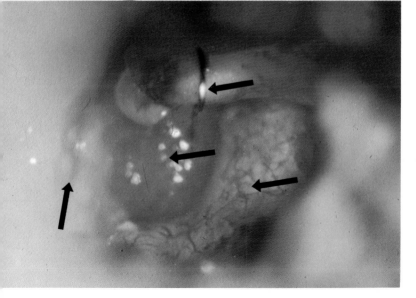

FACIAL PALSY

124 Bell's palsy The commonest cause of facial palsy. It is a lower motor neurone lesion of the facial nerve, of unknown aetiology, involving a loss of movement of facial muscles, usually total, of one side of the face. This includes the muscles of the forehead (with facial paralysis due to an upper motor neurone lesion such as a stroke these muscles continue to function due to cross innervation distal to the cortex). Pain in or around the ear frequently precedes Bell's Palsy and a history of draught on the side of the face may be significant. Bell's Palsy may be recurrent and associated with parotid swelling (Melkersson's syndrome). The aetiology and management of Bell's Palsy is controversial. Oedema of the facial nerve near the stylo-mastoid foramen has been demonstrated but the cause is unknown. Most Bell's palsies recover completely and spontaneously within six weeks. Physiotherapy maintains tone in the facial muscles during recovery, and it is probable that oral steroids in high doses* in the early stage of Bell's improve the prognosis.

Facial palsy may follow skull fracture or facial nerve laceration near the stylo-mastoid foramen, and is also an uncommon complication of middle ear surgery and superficial parotidectomy. An extensive cholesteotoma or middle ear carcinoma may also damage the facial nerve : in the absence of a careful examination of the tympanic membrane such a case may be wrongly diagnosed and treated as a Bell's palsy. All facial palsies should have otological assessment.

Bilateral facial palsy is an interesting rarity. It is the facial assymmetry of facial palsy that is conspicuous and makes the diagnosis obvious : a bilateral facial palsy may not be so readily diagnosed.

Prednisolone 20mgs q.d.s. 5 days
Prednisolone 20mgs t.d.s. 1 day
Prednisolone 20mgs b.d. 1 day
Prednisolone 20mgs o.d. 1 day
Prednisolone 10mgs o.d. 1 day

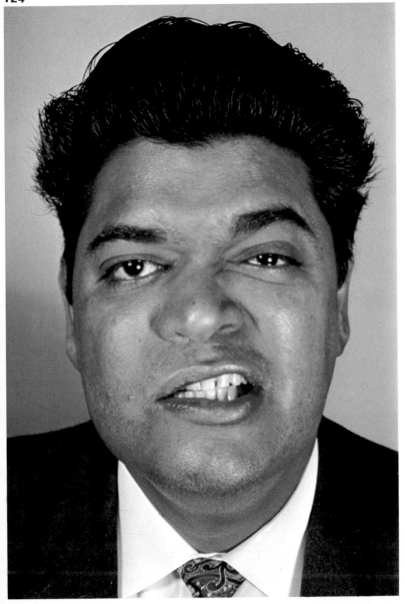

125 & 126   Tests of facial nerve involvement   The level of involvement of the facial nerve in facial palsy can be determined by three tests:

1   Taste (electrogustometry, page 40): if taste is absent or impaired the lesion is proximal to the chorda tympani.

2.   Stapedial reflex (see **20** and **21**, impedance audiometry).

3.   Lachrymation (Schirmer's test, **125**). Litmus paper is placed under the lower lid. If the facial nerve lesion is proximal to, or involves the geniculate ganglion, the tears are reduced.

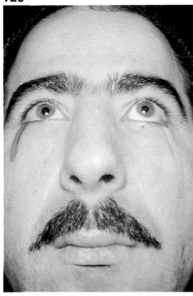

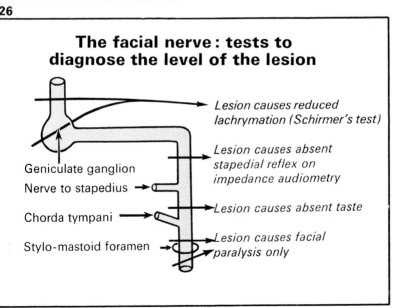

The facial nerve: tests to diagnose the level of the lesion

Geniculate ganglion

Nerve to stapedius →

Chorda tympani →

Stylo-mastoid foramen →

Lesion causes reduced lachrymation (Schirmer's test)

Lesion causes absent stapedial reflex on impedance audiometry

Lesion causes absent taste

Lesion causes facial paralysis only

MICROSURGERY

127 & 128 The middle ear operating microscope   Modern
middle ear surgery has been possible because of the development of the
middle ear operating microscope. This apparatus makes the drum,
ossicles and other middle ear structures easy to manipulate with fine
instruments.

The microscope is either sterilised with a drape (**127**) or an antiseptic,
and a camera and tutor arm can be attached (**128**).

127

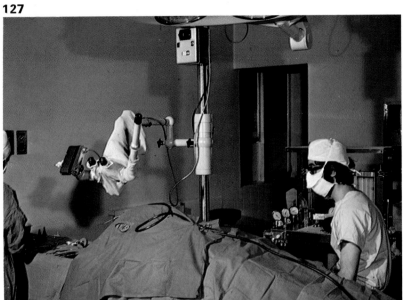

128

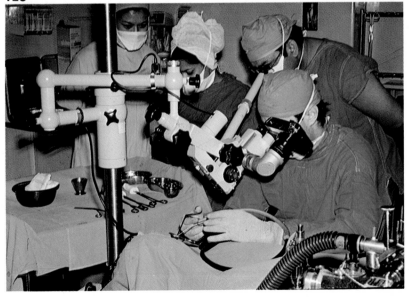

The Nose

DEFORMITIES

129 Congenital deformities Abnormal fusion of the nasal processes (seen here) is uncommon and results in a severe deformity. Congenital atresia of one posterior choana is another congenital deformity and may not present until adult life; a total unilateral obstruction from birth may cause surprisingly little trouble to the patient. If, however, the symptoms are marked the atresia can be treated surgically with removal of the bony obstruction. Bilateral atresia presents as a crisis in early life, and must be remembered as a cause of dyspnoea soon after birth. Metal cannulae are placed through both nasal fossae. If the atresia is membraneous this may suffice, but bony atresia requires later operation.

130 Haemangiomas These are seen in children and are a cosmetic problem. Treatment is deferred, for this lesion may regress before adolescence. If the deformity is gross, removal of the haemangioma with skin grafting to the defect may be necessary: cryosurgery also promises to be effective treatment, but a good cosmetic result is not easily achieved.

129

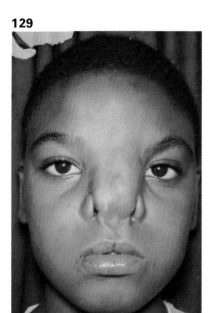

130

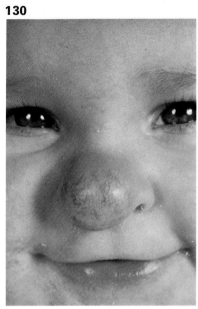

CYSTS

131 & 132   Naso-alveolar cysts   These cysts are constant in their site. Externally, there is flattening of the naso-labial fold and flaring of the alae nasi. In the anterior nares the cyst extends into the floor of the nose and displaces the inferior turbinate upwards.

133   Typical presentation   The naso-alveolar cyst is common in Negroes, and its constant anatomical site makes spot diagnosis possible. Excision via a sublabial incision and enucleation is the treatment. Surgical rupture of the cyst usually means incomplete removal and predisposes to recurrence. *Arrow* indicates 'flaring' of ala.

134   Dermoid   A cystic swelling near the glabella is probably a dermoid; excision is straightforward. The differential diagnosis in childhood is the *nasal glioma*. This unusual nasal tumour is benign and presents either externally or as an intranasal swelling. It is either a completely separate firm tumour, or is connected to the cerebrum through a dehiscence in the cribriform plate. X-rays to exclude an intracranial origin are necessary before a nasal glioma is excised.

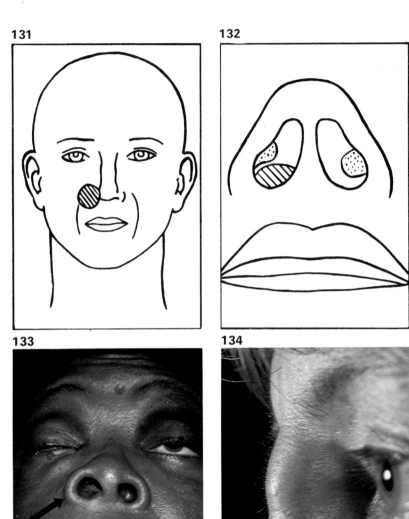

131

132

133

134

ADENOIDS

135 Adenoids A mass of lymphoid tissue shaped like a bunch of bananas, occupies the vault of the post-nasal space in children. If the adenoids are large, nasal obstruction occurs. There is snoring, with purulent rhinorrhoea if there is a secondary sinusitis, and epistaxis. Aural symptoms due to interference with the Eustachian tube also occur, with or without nasal symptoms; there is deafness due to secretory otitis media, or earache from recurrent acute otitis media.

Adenoids normally regress before puberty and adults with large adenoids are rare. If an adult has nasal obstruction due to post-nasal lymphoid tissue, the histology is essential to exclude a lymphosarcoma. Nasal obstruction may occur from birth due to large adenoids, and the baby has difficulty with bottle and breast feeding. It is occasionally necessary to remove these 'congenital adenoids' in toddlers. A conservative attitude should be taken however with removal of adenoids, awaiting natural regression of the lymphoid tissue; only marked nasal and aural symptoms necessitate operation.

136 Lateral x-ray of adenoids The post-nasal space is often difficult or impossible to see in a child and a lateral x-ray shows clearly the size of the adenoids and degree of obstruction. In this x-ray a small airway is present despite a large adenoid shadow.

135

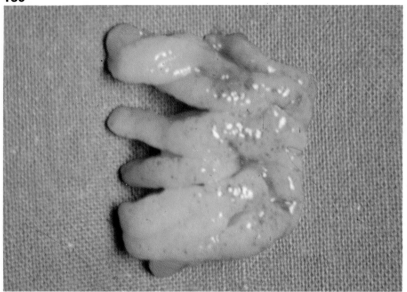

136

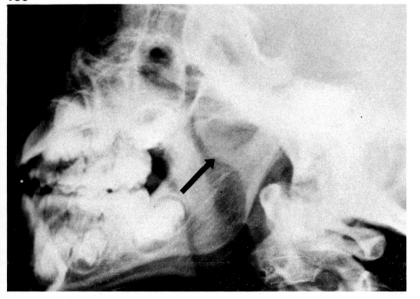

TRAUMA

137   Fractured nose   This common injury only requires treatment if the septum is dislocated or involved in haematoma, or if there is an external deviation of the nose (seen here) of cosmetic concern to the patient. It is important to reduce nasal fractures within two weeks, lest the bones cannot be manipulated and a subsequent rhinoplasty may be necessary. Reduction is therefore carried out either soon after fracture, or is delayed until the oedema, which makes assessment of the deformity difficult, has settled.

Many fractured noses, however, are 'chip' or undisplaced crack injuries with haematoma, and require no treatment.

138   Complete separation of one nasal bone   In this injury there is a deviation of the bones and the x-ray shows a complete separation of one nasal bone. A black eye is a common feature of a fractured nose.

One alarming and unusual complication of a nasal fracture is surgical emphysema of the orbit when the patient blows the nose. This is due to a fracture through the ethmoidal cells and lamina papyracea linking the nasal cavity to the orbit. There is no cause for alarm, and care not to inflate the orbit is followed by spontaneous healing.

A facial injury that has caused a nasal fracture, may also have involved the maxilla and anterior cranial fossa (with C.S.F. rhinorrhoea) and precautions should be taken to exclude such an associated fracture.

137

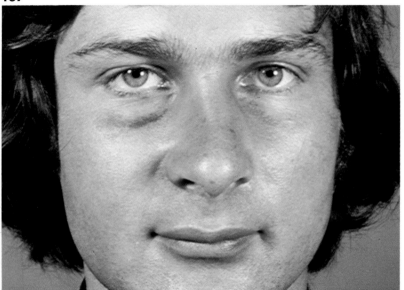

138

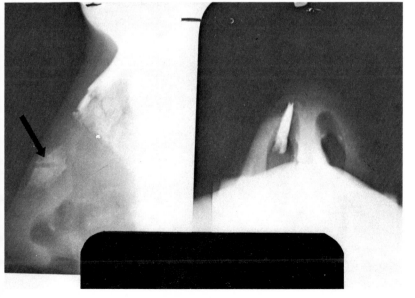

113

139   Complications of a fractured nose   A septal haematoma causes complete nasal obstruction; secondary infection may occur and is characterised by pain. Incision of the septum and drainage is necessary. The patient must be warned *before* operation that a *saddle deformity* (as here) due to lack of septal support may develop following a haematoma. A septal haematoma may also follow surgical correction of a deviated septum (submucous resection).

140   Retraction of the columella   A retraction and loss of tip support of the nose are less usual complications of a septal haematoma.

139

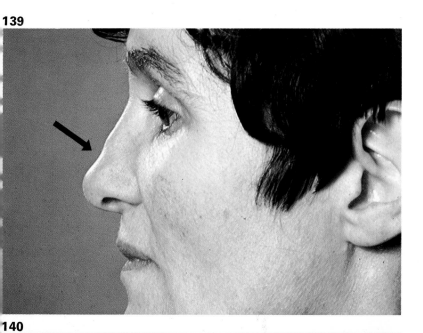

140

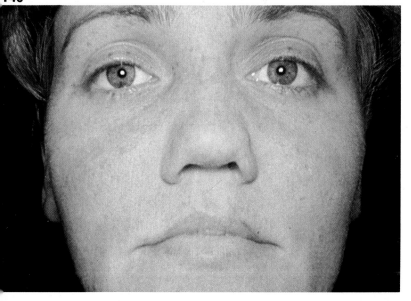

141–144   Rhinoplasty   The appearance of a nose with a congenital or traumatic hump or deviation of the nasal bones can be improved with rhinoplasty (**141, 142**). Bulbous, prominent or depressed tips (**143, 144**) due to alar cartilage changes can also be modified. Incisions for rhinoplasty are within the nasal vestibule and access to the nasal bones, cartilages, and septum is obtained with an intranasal approach.

141

142

143

144

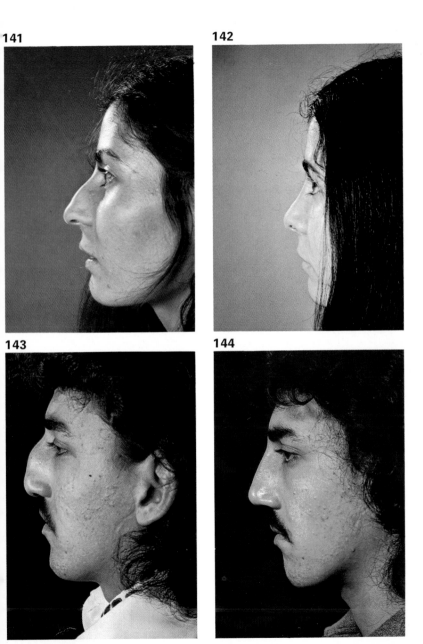

145 Deviated nasal septum A congenital or traumatic disloca-
tion of the septal cartilage into one nasal fossa causes unilateral nasal
obstruction. If the obstruction is marked, or complicated by recurrent
sinusitis, a submucous resection (S.M.R.), or septal reposition is minor
and effective surgery.

146 Septal spur indenting the inferior turbinate A posterior
deviation of the septum can be overlooked, and a vasoconstrictor
applied to the anterior nasal mucous membrane reduces the size of the
turbinates and allows a clear view posteriorly. *Arrow* indicates septal
spur.

147 A posterior septal deviation Such deviations of the vomer
and ethmoid bone show on x-ray (*upper arrow*). Also seen on x-ray is
the *compensatory hypertrophy of the inferior turbinate* on the opposite
side to the deviation (*lower arrow*). It is necessary to reduce this
turbinate when the septum is straightened, lest this nasal fossa will
become obstructed post-operatively.

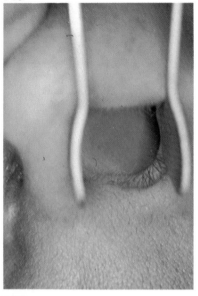

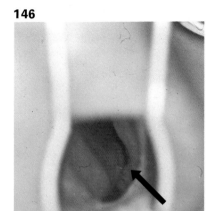

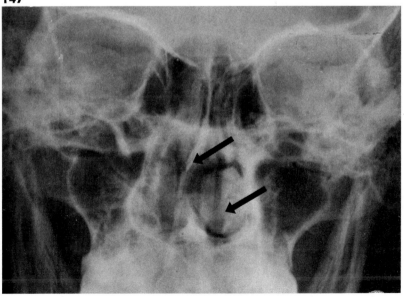

148 A perforation of the nasal septum This may give no symptoms and be a chance finding on examination. Crusting usually occurs, however, and causes nasal obstruction.

149 Prominent blood vessels appearing on the margin of the perforation: these lead to epistaxis. A whistling noise on breathing is another symptom.

Perforations may result from repeated trauma to the septum (e.g. nose picking); chrome workers are susceptible to a septal perichondritis causing a perforation. An inadvertent tear of the nasal mucous membrane on both sides during an S.M.R. operation is another cause of perforation. Destruction of the vomer and ethmoid bone accounts for a posterior septal perforation, and may be due to a gumma.

Surgical repair of a septal perforation, particularly a large one, may not be possible.

148

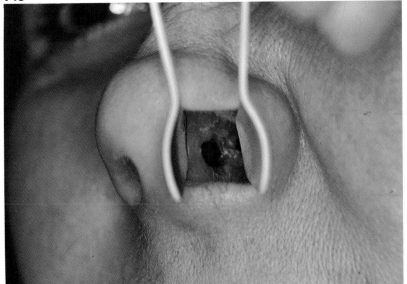

149

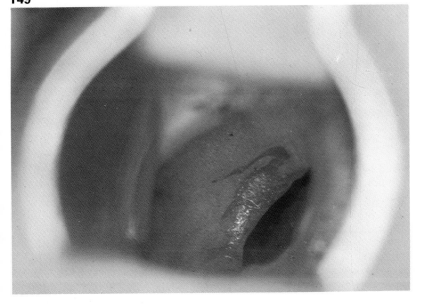

150   A foreign body in the nose causes a unilateral purulent and fetid nasal discharge. A child with these symptoms and a vestibulitis is almost certain to have a foreign body in the nose.

151   Vestibulitis   When nasal discharge and skin involvement affect both nostrils, a vestibulitis (an eczema of the vestibular skin) is the probable diagnosis.

152   Removal of a foreign body   Removal can frequently be managed as an out-patient, when it is necessary to hold the child securely while a probe or hook is placed posterior to the foreign body: forceps frequently push the foreign body posteriorly and should be avoided. A general anaesthetic is necessary if the foreign body is impacted or inaccessable.

A foreign body that is ignored accumulates a calcareous deposit and presents years later as a fetid stony mass—a *rhinolith*.

150

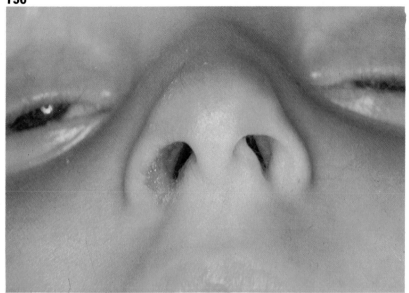

151

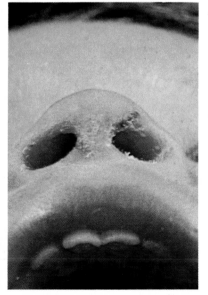

152

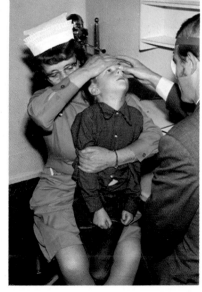

123

INFLAMMATION

153 **Vestibulitis** presents as crusting and irritation in the anterior nares with nasal obstruction. Examination shows excoriated vestibular skin and septal mucous membrane. Rubbing or over-diligent cleaning of the nose by the patient usually causes vestibulitis particularly if, as in this case, the septum is deviated anteriorly and impinges on the lateral wall of the nose. Advice and the use of antibiotic and corticosteroid ointment control vestibulitis. Correction of the septum may be necessary.

154 **Furuncles and cellulitis of the columella** These may spread to involve the skin of the nose and face. Treatment is with systemic penicillin.

153

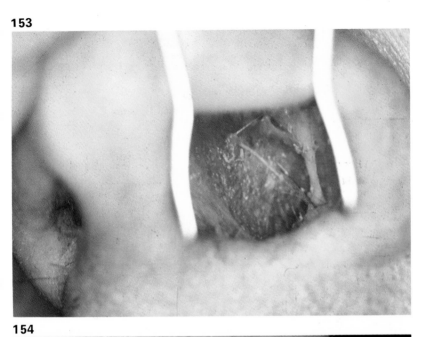

154

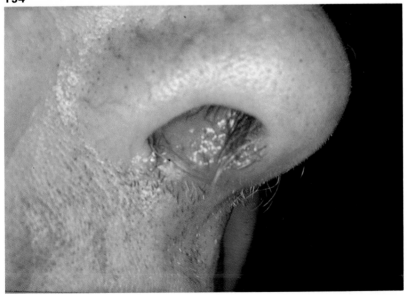

155   Acute rhinitis   In the common cold the nasal mucous membrane is oedematous, so the inferior turbinate abuts against the septum causing obstruction, and there is an excess of mucous causing the running nose. A similar appearance is seen in *nasal allergy*, either 'seasonal hay fever', or perennial allergy, but the oedematous turbinate mucous membrane appears grey rather than red. A persistent purulent nasal discharge usually means that there is a sinusitis.

156   Chronic rhinitis   The turbinate mucous membrane frequently reacts to irritants whether tobacco, excessive use of vasoconstrictor drops or atmospheric irritants, by enlarging. Thickened red inferior turbinates are seen adjacent to the septum limiting the airway. Nasal obstruction, either intermittent or persistent, with a post-nasal discharge of mucous are the symptoms of chronic rhinitis. This is the condition most frequently labelled by the patient as 'catarrh' or 'sinus trouble'. If the changes due to the chronic rhinitis are irreversible, i.e. the nasal obstruction persists when the irritants are removed, it is probable that minor surgery to reduce the turbinates in size will be necessary. Occasionally, oral antihistamines help, but vasoconstrictor drops have no place in the treatment of chronic rhinitis and their constant use is a common cause of this condition (*rhinitis medicamentosa*).

In most inflammatory conditions of the nasal mucous membrane there is an excess of mucous. An atrophy of the mucosa and mucous glands with fetid crusting of wide nasal fossae is, however, seen with *atrophic rhinitis.* This is uncommon and idiopathic: it may be an isolated nasal condition or part of Wegener's granuloma or disseminated lupus erythematosus. There is also a phase of atrophic nasal crusting in rhinoscleroma.

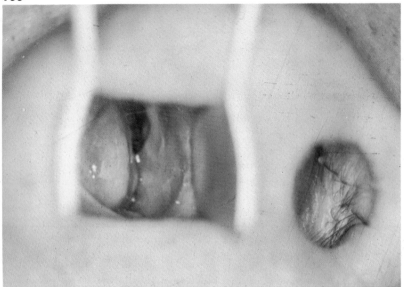

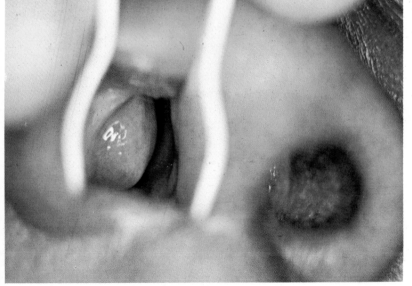

157 & 158   Acute maxillary sinusitis   This is a common compli-cation of a head cold. Apical infection of the teeth related to the antrum, or an oro-antral fistula following dental extraction also cause maxillary sinusitis, as may trauma with bleeding into the antrum or barotrauma. Frontal or facial pain may be referred to the upper teeth. Nasal obstruction and purulent rhinorrhoea are the other symptoms. The antrum is *opaque* on x-ray, as seen here, and dull on transillumination. There is tenderness over the sinus but swelling is rare. Pus is seen issuing from the middle meatus (**158**).

Acute infection may less commonly affect the ethmoid, frontal and sphenoid sinuses. Systemic antibiotics, a vasoconstrictor spray or drops, and inhalations are usually curative for acute sinusitis. A persis-tent maxillary sinusitis, however, requires an antral washout.

159   An antral washout   This involves inserting a trocar and can-nula under the inferior turbinate, and puncturing the lateral wall of the nose through the maxillary process of the thin inferior turbinate bone, to enter the antrum. Water is irrigated through the cannula and the pus emerges through the maxillary ostium. *An acutely infected maxillary sinus must not be washed out*, until medical treatment has controlled the acute phase; cavernous sinus thrombosis remains a danger. The bad reputation that antral washout has for pain is not justified if a good local anaesthetic and gentle technique are used.

Recurrent attacks of acute maxillary sinusitis may require operation. A permanent intranasal opening into the antrum is made either in the middle or inferior meatus (intranasal antrostomy). This operation is also effective for those cases of acute sinusitis that fail to respond to con-servative treatment and antral washouts.

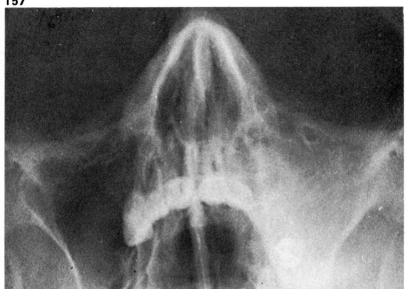

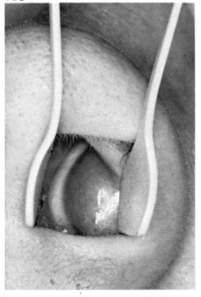

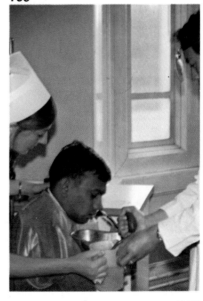

160   Orbital cellulitis   Complications of acute sinusitis confined to the antrum are rare. A severe maxillary sinusitis, however, usually involves the ethmoid and frontal sinuses. Infection spreading via the lamina papyracea or floor of the frontal sinus leads to an *orbital cellulitis.*

161   Orbital abscess   Such an abscess, requiring external drainage, may form. Meningitis or brain abscess may also follow spread of infection from the roof of the ethmoid, frontal or sphenoid sinus to the anterior cranial fossa. Infection associated with a rapidly growing neoplasm, such as a rhabdomyosarcoma, is the differential diagnosis in the case illustrated.

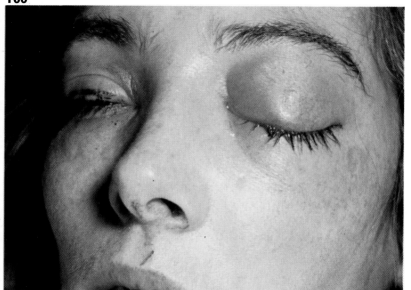

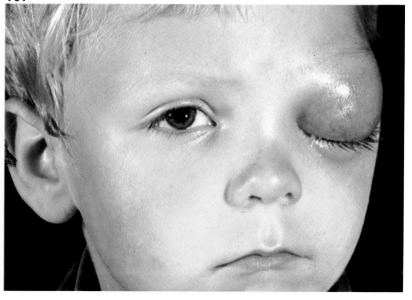

Chronic sinusitis This may develop from incomplete resolution of an acute infection. The onset may, however, be insidious and secondary to nasal obstruction (e.g. due to a deviated septum, nasal polyps, or, in children, to enlarged adenoids). Apical infection of the teeth related to the antra can also cause chronic sinusitis.

Purulent rhinorrhoea, nasal obstruction and headache are the main symptoms of chronic sinusitis. Pus in the middle meatus with opacity of the sinus are confirmatory of infection. Pus confined to the antrum rarely gives complications, but often there is spread of infection to the ethmoids and frontal sinuses. It is not common for frontal and ethmoidal sinusitis to occur without maxillary sinusitis. Pus in the frontal and ethmoid sinus may, as with acute infections, spread to involve the orbit and brain. Obstruction of the sinus ostium may lead to an encysted collection of mucous within the sinus—a mucocele.

162–164 A mucocele The frontal sinus is commonly affected and erosion of the roof of the orbit leads to orbital displacement downwards and laterally. Proptosis also occurs and is best confirmed by examination from above (**163**). The frontal sinus wall may be eroded both posteriorly and anteriorly. An eroded anterior wall results in a fluctuant swelling on the forehead (**164**). In this case there is also orbital displacement and proptosis.

165 Lateral displacement of the orbit This occurs with a mucocele arising in the ethmoid sinus and is usually accompanied by swelling at the medial canthus. In this case the mucocele is infected—*a pyocele*.

162

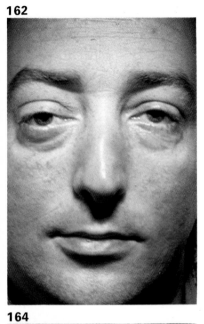

163

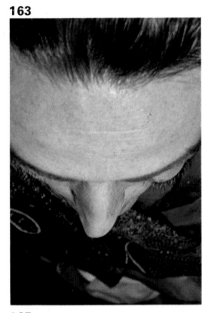

164

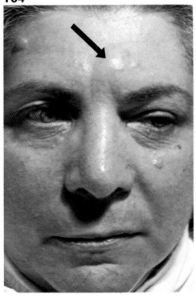

165

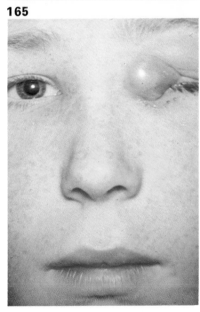

133

166 & 167   The Caldwell-Luc operation   Chronic   maxillary sinusitis may require the Caldwell-Luc operation in which the antrum is opened with a sublabial antrostomy, the antral mucous membrane is removed, and an intranasal antrostomy made. If the ethmoid cells are involved,   they   can   be   removed   with   this   approach   (transantral ethmoidectomy). Chronic maxillary sinusitis tends to have a reputation for being difficult to treat, with recurrence being common. This is not justified, for treatment is usually curative.

Chronic frontal sinusitis may also require surgery and is treated with an external approach. Obliteration of the sinus with a fat graft, or enlarging the fronto-nasal duct are the two current operations.

166

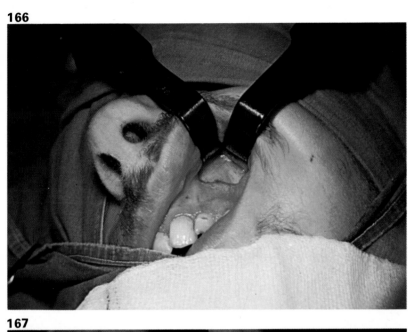

167

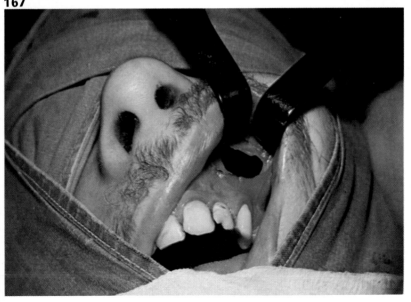

168 & 169   Maxillary sinus x-rays   In acute and chronic maxillary sinusitis fluid may be seen on x-ray. It is essential if a *fluid level* (**168**) is seen for a tilted view (**169**) to be taken to confirm the presence of fluid. A thickened and rather straight mucous membrane may look like a fluid level, as may a bony shadow if the x-ray is wrongly angled. Fluid levels are also seen in the frontal sinuses.

168

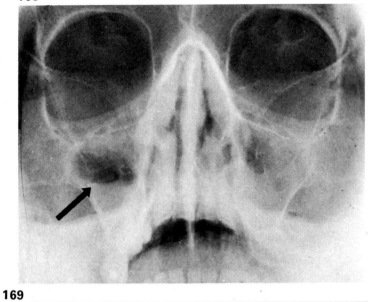

169

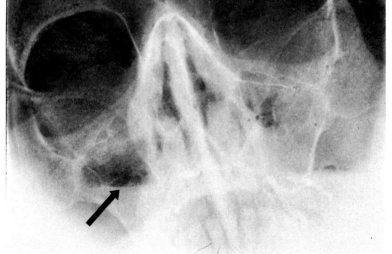

170   Nasal polyps   These are a common cause of nasal obstruction and may cause anosmia. They are benign and do not present with bleeding. Examination shows a grey pendulous opalescent swelling arising from the ethmoid. A polyp is very different in appearance to the red inferior turbinate adjacent to it.

Polyps may be solitary or multiple, often extending from the nasal vestibule to the posterior choana. They are usually bilateral. If ignored, nasal polyps may become extremely large, causing expansion of the nasal bones and alae nasi. A nasal polyp which is ulcerated and bleeds is probably malignant.

Nasal polyps result from a distension of an area of nasal mucous membrane with intercellular fluid. They are due to a hypersensitivity reaction in the mucous membrane, but may also result from sinus infection. Obstruction of the sinuses by polyps may, however, lead to a secondary sinusitis, and a sinus x-ray is a routine investigation.

Extensive or recurrent polyps require removal under general anaesthetic but smaller polyps can be removed in Out-Patients under local anaesthetic.

171   Polyp in the oropharynx   Large posterior polyps can extend below the soft palate and present in the oropharynx.

A solitary polyp from one posterior choana is almost certainly an *antrochoanal polyp* (*arrowed*), but a rare vascular polyp which should be remembered in the differential diagnosis is the *angiofibroma of male puberty.*

172   Enlarged posterior ends of the inferior turbinates   These turbinates may enlarge in chronic rhinitis (and in nasal allergy) to produce a large polypoid mass obstructing the posterior choanae (*arrowed*). If these cannot be seen with the post-nasal mirror, they are demonstrated on the lateral x-ray.

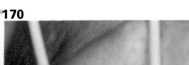

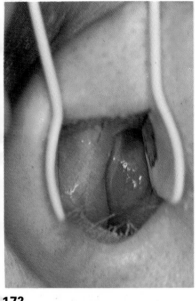

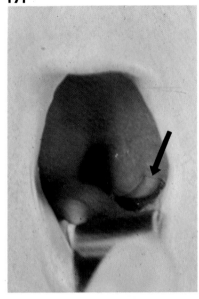

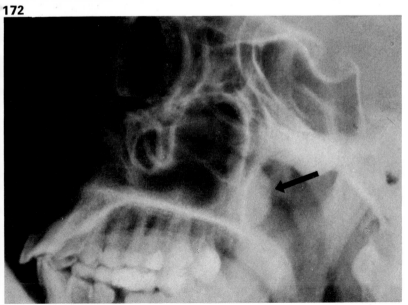

173   Antrochoanal polyp   This is a special type of nasal polyp occurring in adolescents and young adults. Unilateral nasal obstruction is caused by a grey single polyp seen in the post-nasal space. The maxillary sinus is opaque on x-ray.

174   Antrochoanal polyp   This type of polyp, which arises from the antral mucosa, extrudes through the ostium to fill the posterior nasal fossa and post-nasal space.   It frequently becomes extremely large and extends below the soft palate.   Removal of the polyp from its origin in the antrum through a sublabial antrostomy approach is necessary. The polyp is dumb-belled in shape with a pedicle connecting the nasal and antral portions. Intranasal removal is invariably followed by recurrence but may be necessary in early adolescence if the permanent dentition is endangered by a sublabial antrostomy. *Top arrow* shows polyp removed from antrum; *second arrow* shows polyp from nasal fossa; *third arrow* indicates polyp from post-nasal space; *bottom arrow* indicates polyp that has extended into oropharynx.

175   Aspiration from the antrum   This shows straw coloured fluid, and is a reliable diagnostic test for an antrochoanal polyp.

173

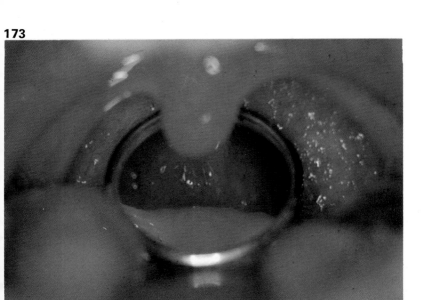

174

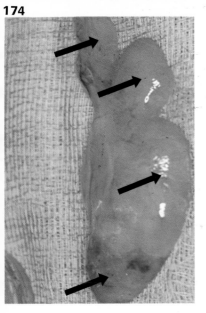

175

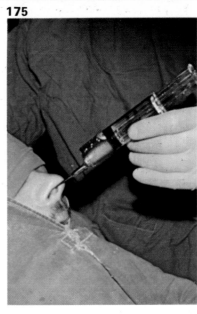

176 Epistaxis Anteriorly on the septum there is an anastamosis of several arteries (the sphenopalatine, the greater palatine, the superio labial and the anterior ethmoidal). This site is called Little's or Kiesselbach's plexus and is the commonest site of nose bleeds.

There are numerous causes of epistaxis. Some such as trauma and acute inflammatory nasal conditions are obvious and common, but the more serious local and general causes must not be overlooked. Diagnosis must follow control of the epistaxis. Hypertension and blood dyscrasia are important general causes, and neoplasms and telangiectasia may be underlying local factors.

177 Cautery If epistaxis is recurrent, cautery (which is painless with local anaesthetic) to the bleeding point is necessary either with the galvano-cautery or with a chemical (e.g. trichloracetic acid or silve nitrate). Trichloracetic acid used in this case causes the bleeding site in Little's plexus to become white. Care must be taken to avoid the chemical running onto the skin of the vestibule or face as scarring will result. A topical anaesthetic is applied to the nasal mucous membrane in Little's Area for galvano-cautery but with silver nitrate and trichloracetic acid, no anaesthetic is needed and the procedure is painless, providing the vestibular skin is not touched.

178 Bleeding polyp Occasionally, a small vascular sessile polyp is seen on the septum (haemangioma) which is the cause of severe recurrent bleeds. Treatment is excision, or cautery if the lesion is small.

Epistaxis from the anterior septum may be profuse and alarming but firm sustained pressure on the nares is invariably effective. Posterior epistaxis from the sphenopalatine artery may be very severe and difficult to manage. Nasal packing is needed to control the acute phase and ligation of the maxillary or external carotid artery is necessary if bleeding is persistent or severe. The terminal branch of the anterior ethmoidal artery may be the site of bleeding superiorly in the nose, particularly with nasal fractures : this vessel too may require ligation.

176

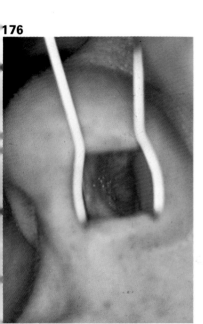

177

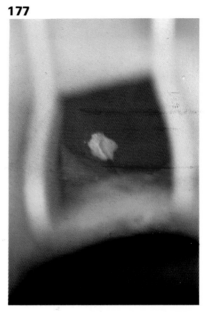

178

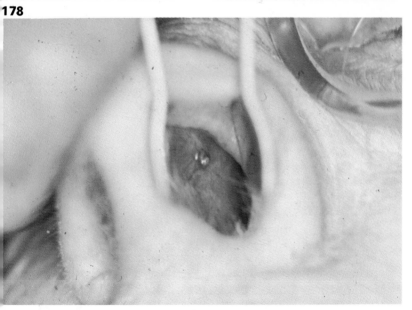

NEOPLASMS

Malignant nasal tumours   A nasal polyp that does not appear grey and opalescent should arouse suspicion, as should a polyp that bleeds spontaneously. A solid looking hyperaemic polyp may be a transitional cell papilloma. Granulation tissue in the nose may be malignant granuloma or carcinoma, and biopsy of any suspicious nasal lesion is necessary

179   A pigmented polyp may be a malignant melanoma.

180, 181 & 182   Carcinomas of the antrum or ethmoid   These may extend not only into the nasal fossa and cheek (**180**) but may present in the oral cavity (**181**) appearing as a dental lesion. The antrum is opaque on x-ray with evidence of *bony destruction* (*arrowed*, **182**)

Prognosis when radiotherapy is followed by maxillectomy is quite good for an early maxillary carcinoma, but poor when there is extensive invasion. Exenteration of the orbit with maxillectomy is necessary when the eye is involved, but carcinoma with posterior spread to the base of the skull is inoperable. The use of cytotoxic drugs (e.g. methotrexate) either orally or combined with intra-arterial infusion results in regression in some of these paranasal sinus neoplasms and is a further line of treatment.

179

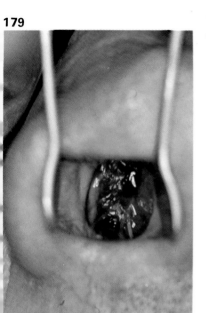

180

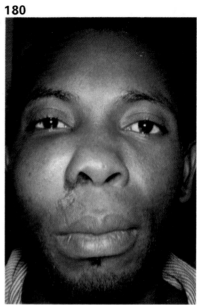

181

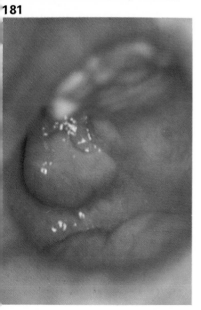

182

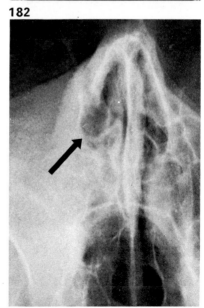

183   Carcinoma of the external nose   This is uncommon. Wide surgical excision with forehead reconstructive rhinoplasty, or less commonly radiotherapy are the available treatments.

184   Carcinoma of the septum and columella

185   Chronic inflammation of the nose   Lupus vulgaris is now rare. It presents as a chronic ulcer of the nasal vestibule extending onto the face. The differential diagnosis of inflammatory ulceration anteriorly in the nose includes sarcoidosis which may also cause destruction of the ala. Biopsy is necessary for the diagnosis.

186   The effects of lupus vulgaris   Lupus, if ignored, is destructive to the skin and cartilage of the alae nasi and septum.

183

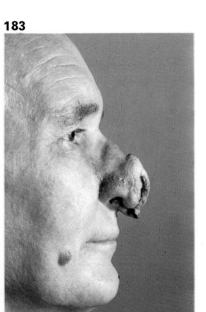

184

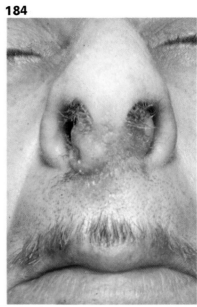

185

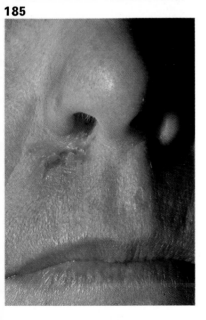

186

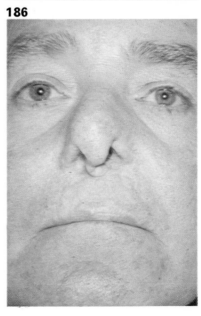

187　Carcinoma of the nasopharynx　This is uncommon in most countries but has an unexplained high incidence in the Far East, particularly in China, and East Africa.

There are many presenting symptoms (**187**). As the posterior choanae are large, nasal obstruction is not common with ulcerated carcinomas, which tend to present with symptoms of nerve involvement or secretory otitis media due to interference with the Eustachian tube. Lympho-sarcomas and papilliferous carcinomas do however cause obstruction. Carcinoma invades the skull base involving the Vth, VIth and Vidian (Pterygoid) nerves, and may cause headache by invasion of the dura. The nasopharynx is a relatively concealed site and presentation of carcinoma is commonly late, with a cervical node metastasis.

The treatment is with radiotherapy and the prognosis is not good with about a 30% five year survival rate.

Symptoms of carcinoma of nasopharynx

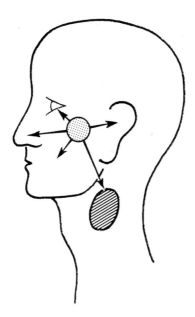

Nasal
  Obstruction
  Sanguineous discharge

Neurological
  Facial pain or
  numbness due
  to involvement
  of Vth nerve

Ear
  Deafness due to
  secretory otitis media
  Pain

Eye
  Proptosis due to direct
  spread to orbit
  Diplopia due to involvement of VIth nerve

Neck
  Neck mass due to
  cervical metastasis

The Pharynx and Larynx

THE OROPHARYNX

188 A mucocele of the lip Mucoceles are cystic, non-tender swellings presenting on the lips or in the oral cavity. They result from extravasation of mucous from a mucous gland into the surrounding tissue. Treatment is excision which is not always easy because of the extremely thin wall, and simple marsupialisation is often adequate.

189 Lip ulcers Lip ulceration has numerous causes, either traumatic, inflammatory, or neoplastic: the provisional diagnosis can be made from this history and type of ulcer. Biopsy is necessary to confirm the diagnosis. This lesion is a *pyogenic granuloma.*

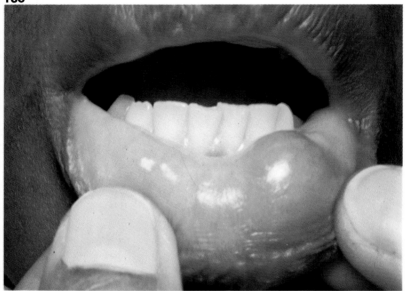

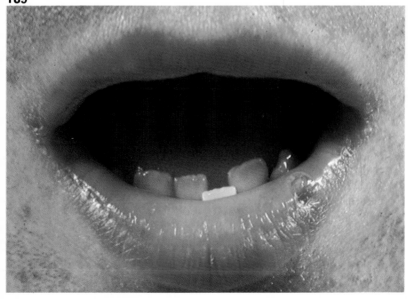

190   Hyperkeratosis may extend from the angle of the mouth along the occlusal plane of the teeth and is commonly a dental problem: it may be self-induced due to nervous cheek-biting. It is often the result of persistent trauma to the mucous membrane. When occurring in a site not exposed to trauma, e.g. the retromolar fossa, it should arouse suspicion that the mucosal change may be malignant and a biopsy is necessary.

191   Angular stomatitis   This occurs with the type of dental hyperkeratosis shown in **190**, but it may also be part of a syndrome: the Plummer-Vinson or Patterson-Brown-Kelly Syndrome. Glossitis, apparent in this picture, and hypochromic anaemia are associated with a post-cricoid lesion, either a web or a carcinoma. This syndrome occurs almost exclusively in women.

190

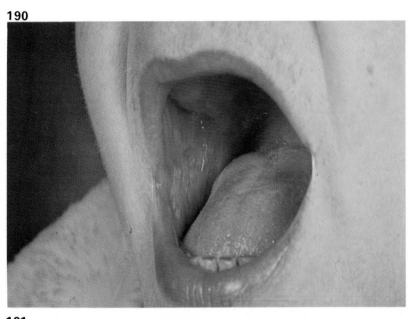

191

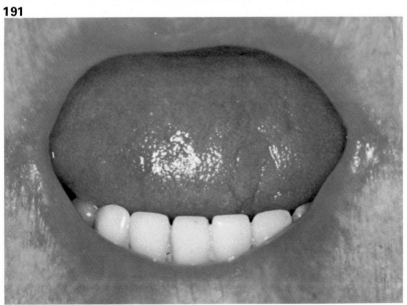

153

192 The torus palatinus The bony hard midline palatal swelling can be diagnosed confidently by its characteristics. It is a common finding and only requires removal if it interferes with the fitting of a denture. Similar bony swellings occur less commonly on the lingual surface of the lower alveolus opposite the premolars (torus mandibularis).

193 Ectopic pleomorphic adenoma A palatal swelling which is not bony and hard may be a fissural cyst if midline, but if placed to one side (as here), it is almost certainly a tumour of one of the minor salivary glands. Biopsy is necessary. It is frequently a pleomorphic adenoma, but may be a cylindroma or a more malignant salivary tumour.

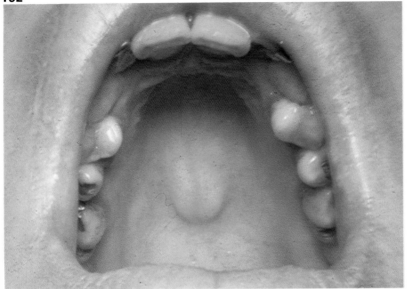

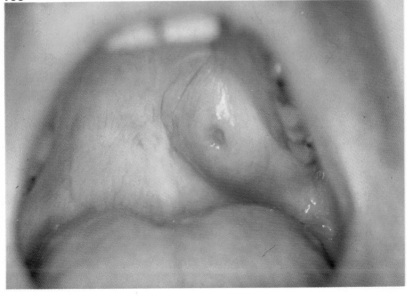

194 & 195   Aphthous ulcers   An area of white superficial ulceration is surrounded by a hyperaemic mucous membrane. These commonly occur in crops of two or more and heal spontaneously in about one week. They are acutely tender and affect the non-keratinised oral mucous membrane. Although there is no induration on palpation, the histological inflammatory changes are not superficial and may extend into the underlying muscle.

Hydrocortisone pellets to suck, or triamcinolone with orobase ointment applied to the ulcer are the most effective present treatment to relieve the pain. As the aetiology of these extremely common ulcers remains unknown, treatment is empirical.

196   Trauma from a denture   This may be an initiating factor, as may any minor trauma to the mucous membrane in a person susceptible to aphthous ulcers.

194

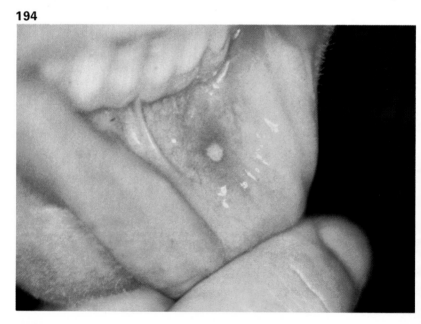

195

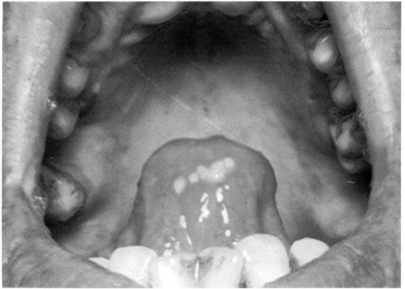

196

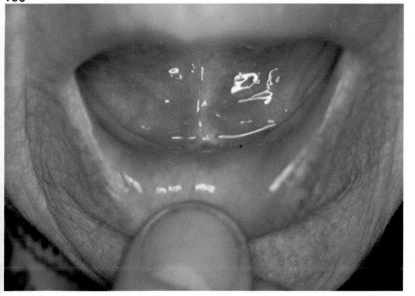

197 Possible salivary calculus An ulcer in the region of the orifice of the parotid duct suggests a possible salivary calculus.

198 Solitary aphthous ulcer This ulcer (*periadenitis mucosa necrotica recurrens*) looks similar to a simple aphthous ulcer, and is the same histologically, but it behaves differently. It is less common, larger, persists for several weeks or months and may leave a scar; it occurs in more varied sites affecting the soft palate and even the pyriform fossa, where it presents with severe dysphagia. Carbenoxylone ('Bioral') is used topically for the lesions in the oral cavity.

199 Multiple oral ulcers These may be the herpetiform type of aphthous ulceration. They may, however, be due to a blood dyscrasia; if the ulcers are crusted and haemorrhagic (seen here) the condition is either erythema multiforme or pemphigus. In this instance an iritis and genital ulceration were present (Behçet's syndrome). High doses of systemic steroids are usually needed to control this type of severe ulceration. The snail-tract ulcers of secondary syphilis must also be remembered in the differential diagnosis of oral ulceration.

197

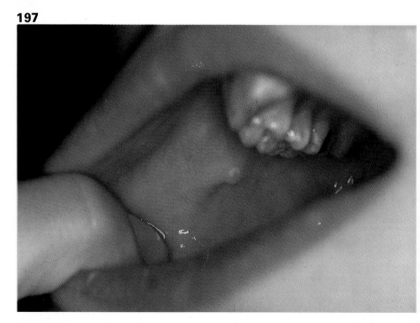

198

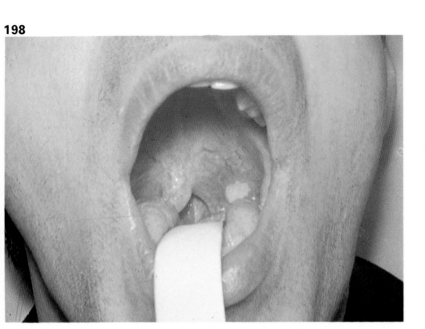

199

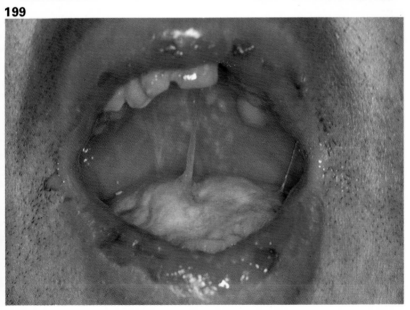

THE TONGUE

200 'Tongue tie' This is due to a short frenulum linguae, and apart from the defect of being unable to protrude the tongue, the patient is almost always symptom-free. Speech defects can rarely be attributed to tongue-tie necessitating division of the frenulum. Division is carried out under general anaesthetic and a suture may be required: a 'snick' of the frenulum with scissors in Out-Patients is inadequate treatment.

201 & 202 Geographic tongue (benign migratory glossitis) There are smooth areas with no filiform papillae. These areas vary in site on the tongue, and the appearance may concern the patient. It is, however, a condition of no significance requiring no treatment other than reassurance.

200

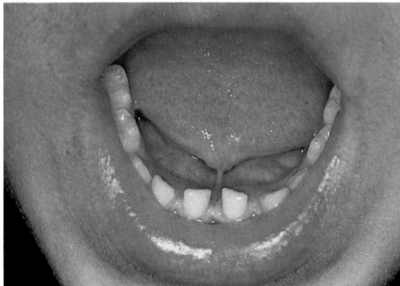

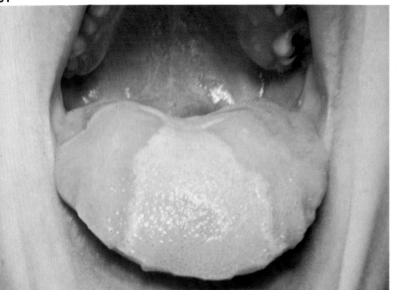

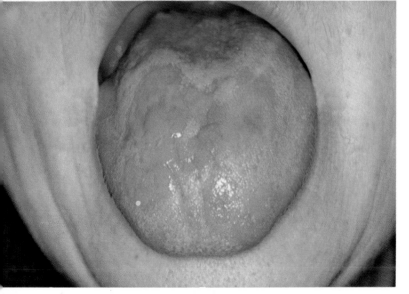

203   Black hairy tongue   Patients not infrequently regard the appearance of their tongue as an index of their general health and are concerned to see a brown-black staining. This may be fungal (Aspergillus niger) and related to prolonged antibiotic therapy, but is frequently a chance finding with no other pathology than hypertrophy of the filiform papillae. Tobacco may be a cause. Scraping and cleaning of the tongue temporarily improves the appearance, but is unnecessary for this condition is harmless.

204   Haemangiomas of the tongue   These may be chance findings and are usually innocuous. If large and giving rise to bleeding, cryosurgery is the most effective present treatment.

203

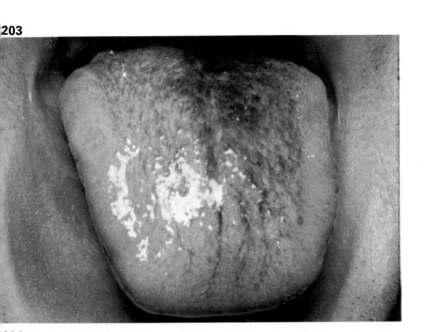

204

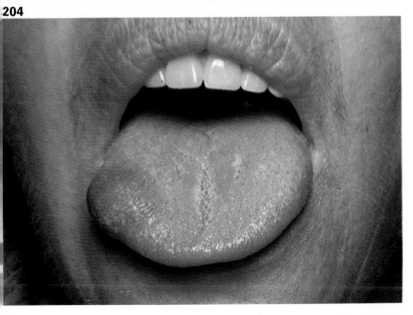

205   The ranula is a mucocele occurring in the floor of the mouth. A blue colour and the profunda vein stretched across the surface are characteristic. This ranula may extend into the tissues of the floor of the mouth and neck (plunging ranula). Total surgical removal is difficult because of the thin wall, and marsupialisation, as with the lip lesion (page 150), is adequate treatment.

206   Lingual thyroid   Developmental anomalies in the thyroid gland may result in thyroid tissue remaining at the foramen caecum or in the thyroglossal tract. The symptom-free swelling at the base of this tongue is thyroid tissue, and was shown on a radio-active iodine scan to be active. No thyroid gland was palpable in the neck and there was no iodine uptake other than at the base of the tongue. This lingual thyroid was, therefore, this patient's only active thyroid tissue.

205

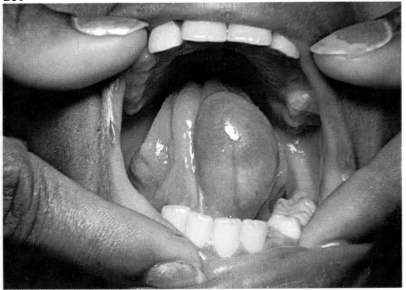

206

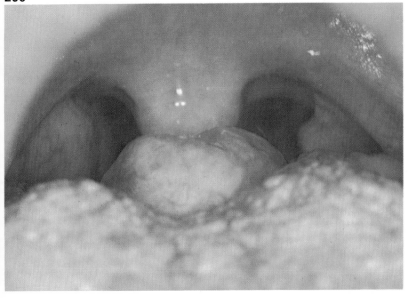

165

207   Tongue ulceration   The site and type of tongue ulcers give the provisional diagnosis: a marginal ulcer with a raised edge is probably a carcinoma; an ulcer on the dorsum with a punched-out margin may be a gumma. Tuberculosis may be the cause of a tender ulcer on the tip of the tongue, in a country where tuberculosis is prevalent. These clinical findings are only guides, however, and biopsy of this ulcer on the dorsum showed it to be a solitary aphthous ulcer (see **198**).

208   Median rhomboid glossitis   This rare anomaly results from failure of the lateral halves of the tongue to fuse posteriorly, leaving the tuberculum impar in the midline. A smooth red, usually symptom-free area persists.

207

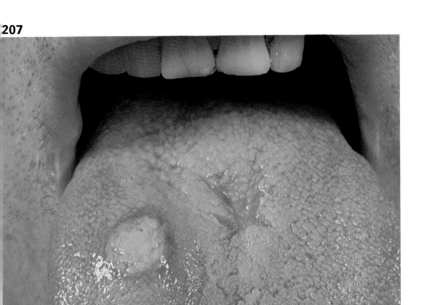

208

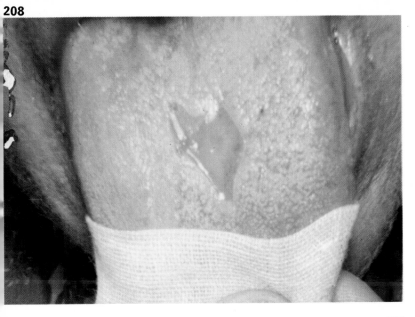

209 Carcinoma of the tongue   This usually occurs on the margin, or from the extension of an ulcer of the floor of the mouth (as shown here). Biopsy of this proliferative ulcer showed squamous cell carcinoma. Partial glossectomy in continuity with a neck dissection, or radiotherapy are the current treatments.

210 Leucoplakia   This is precarcinomatous on the tongue. It may be secondary to dental or dietary irritation. Leucoplakia is also characteristic of tertiary syphilis, and the tongue is a site where the spirochaete predisposes to carcinoma. Leucoplakia, particularly with no apparent underlying traumatic cause, should be biopsied to exclude carcinoma.

209

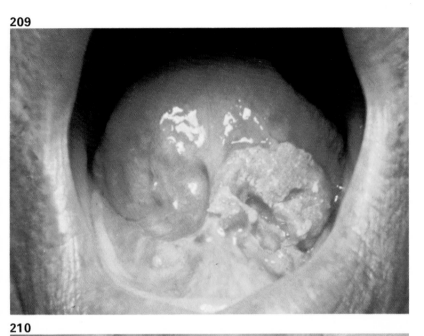

210

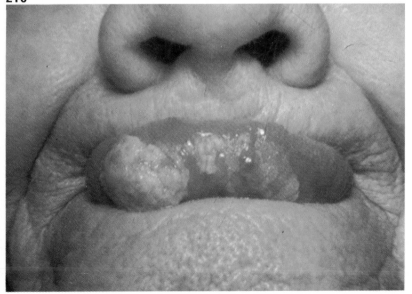

211 Hypoglossal nerve paralysis Initially there is fibrillation and later atrophy of the muscles on one side of the tongue. The tongue deviates on protrusion to the side of the nerve palsy. A destructive lesion in the region of the jugular foramen may extend to involve the hypoglossal nerve as it emerges from the nearby anterior condylar foramen. This paralysis of the tongue shows wrinkling due to fibrillation, and is due to a glomus jugulare tumour, which had also damaged the cranial nerves that emerge through the jugular foramen (IX, X, and XI).

The hypoglossal nerve, if involved with cervical metastases, may be sectioned in the course of a radical neck dissection.

212 Tongue atrophy and deviation This tongue demonstrates the muscle atrophy, and deviation on protrusion.

211

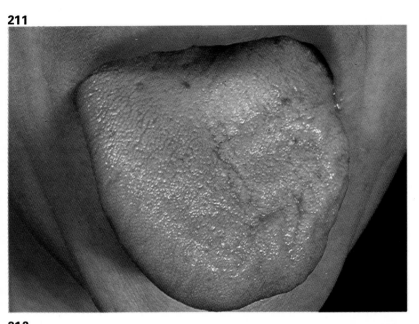

212

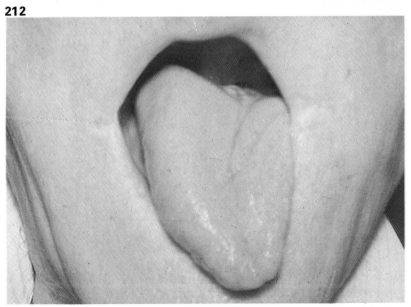

THE FAUCES AND THE TONSILS

213 **Bifid uvula** A common minor congenital deformity of the palate. It is of little significance, but it may be associated with a submucous palatal cleft.

214–217 **Papillomas** These occur on the uvula (**214**), the fauces (**215**) and the tonsil (**216**). The patient often notices these papillomas when looking at his throat, or they are found at medical examination: symptoms are uncommon. They are usually pedunculated and are easily and painlessly removable in Out-Patients. They should be sent for histology to exclude a squamous carcinoma. If ignored a papilloma may cause symptoms on account of size (**217**).

213

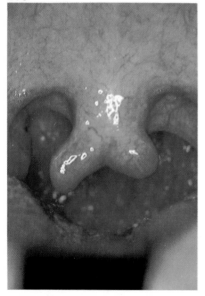

214

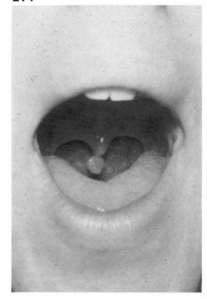

215

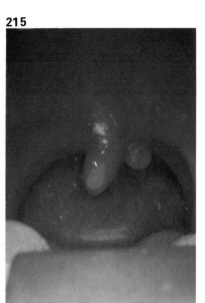

216

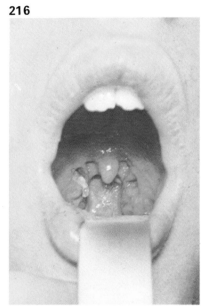

217

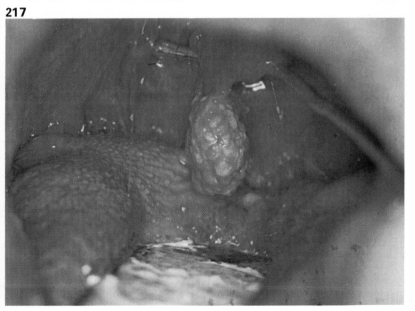

218 & 219   Tonsil size   There is no recognised 'normal' size for a tonsil; it is, therefore, arguable whether tonsils can be described as 'enlarged'. The apparent size of the tonsil can be altered considerably when the tongue is protruded forcibly. This child, whose oropharynx looks normal with the tongue slightly protruded, can make the tonsils meet in the midline with maximum protrusion of the tongue.

220 & 221   Tonsil size affected by tongue depressor   The tongue depressor also alters the apparent size of the tonsils. If the tongue is firmly depressed the patient gags and the tonsils meet in the midline.

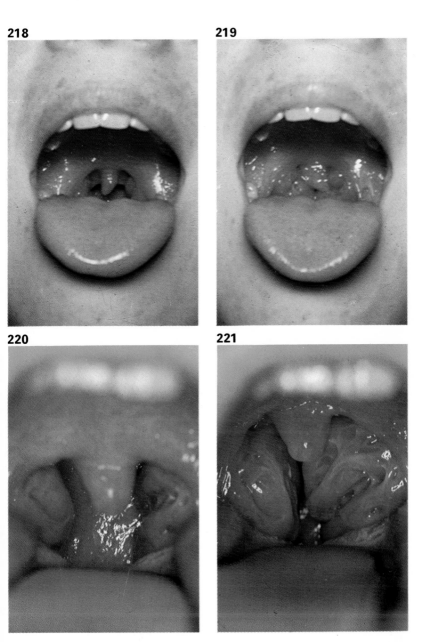

222   Tonsils meeting in the midline   It is, however, unusual for the tonsils to meet in the midline. Lymphoid tissue of this bulk may, particularly during an acute tonsillitis, cause respiratory obstruction and severe dysphagia.

223   Lateral x-ray of tonsils   The tonsils and adenoids show on lateral x-ray and the soft tissue shadow helps in assessing the degree of obstruction that the lymphoid tissue may be causing. The lingual tonsil is unusually large in mongols and contributes to their characteristic bulky tongue.

224   Unilateral tonsil enlargement   A tonsil can be described as 'large' when compared to the other tonsil. A conspicuously large tonsil in the absence of acute inflammation is an important finding suggesting either a *chronic quinsy* or a *lymphosarcoma*. A persistently enlarged tonsil should therefore be removed for histology.

222

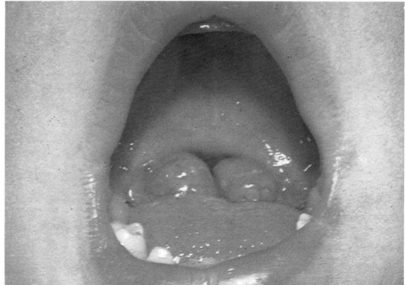

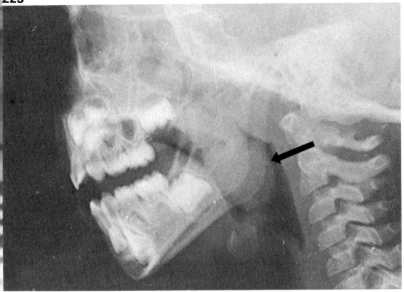

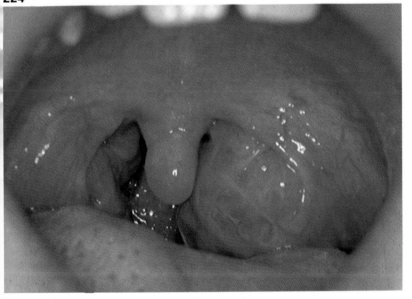

225 A tonsil carcinoma This presents as an indurated ulcer, rather than a diffuse enlargement, and causes pain and otalgia. The biopsy is taken from the ulcer margin. The five year survival following radiotherapy is about 20%.

226 Simulated tonsil enlargement A tonsil may appear to be enlarged by *medial displacement* from a *parapharyngeal swelling* and careful examination of the fauces ensures that the correct diagnosis is made. It is possible to biopsy a normal tonsil, and realise later that medial displacement is simulating enlargement. In this case the parapharyngeal mass is an internal carotid aneurysm: the initial diagnosis in casualty was a quinsy—a dangerous error if followed by incision. Other more common parapharyngeal swellings are tumours of the deep lobe of the parotid gland, chemodectomas, neurofibromata and enlargement of the parapharyngeal lymph nodes.

225

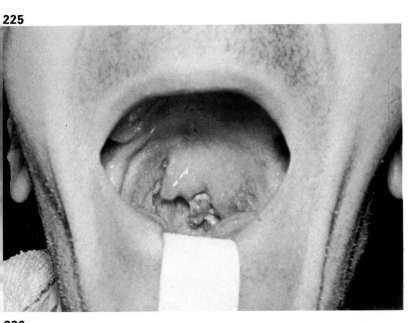

226

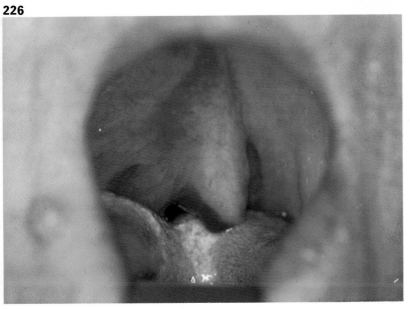

227 & 228 Keratosis pharyngeus Yellow spicules due to hyperkeratinized areas of epithelium are sometimes extensive over the tonsil and lingual tonsil. It is usually a chance finding, and it is important in diagnosis to probe the tonsil to be certain that these yellow areas are not exudate. No treatment is required for this condition unless it is associated with tonsillitis.

229 Retention cysts These are common on the tonsil and appear as sessile yellow swellings. If small, they can be ignored and although symptoms are uncommon, a concern by the patient or a sensation of a lump in the throat, may call for surgical removal.

230 Supratonsillar cleft This recess near the superior pole of the tonsil tends, if large, to collect debris. A mass of yellow fetid material can be extruded from the tonsil with pressure, and discomfort or halitosis are symptoms with which this condition may present. Tonsillectomy may be necessary. The E.N.T. surgeon, however, must beware of tonsillectomy for halitosis. Although dental or gastric pathology may cause this symptom, as may a pharyngeal pouch, the symptom may be imagined by the patient, or in the mind of the other person complaining about the halitosis.

227

228

229

230

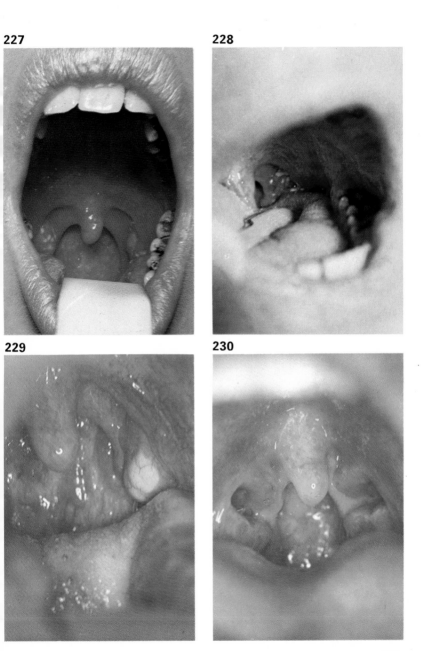

231, 232 & 233   Acute tonsillitis   This condition is characterised by sore throat, dysphagia, and pyrexia. The appearance of the tonsils varies: an obviously purulent exudate covering the tonsils is common and is either diffuse (**231**) or punctate (**232**). An apparently less severely infected throat, with only hyperaemia of the tonsils (**233**) may however be associated with severe symptoms. The tonsillar lymph nodes near the angle of the mandible are large and tender.

With acute tonsillitis the exudate and hyperaemia are centered on the tonsils: in an acute pharyngitis, as may be associated with a head cold, the mucous membrane of the entire oropharynx is hyperaemic. The gonococcus may cause acute pharyngitis and a throat swab must be placed in Stewart's medium for laboratory examination if this infection is suspected. The throat swab in acute tonsillitis commonly grows the haemolytic streptococcus, and a five-day course of oral penicillin (often supplemented with an initial intramuscular injection) is invariably curative. An analgesic may also be needed, but lozenges and gargles are usually unnecessary.

231

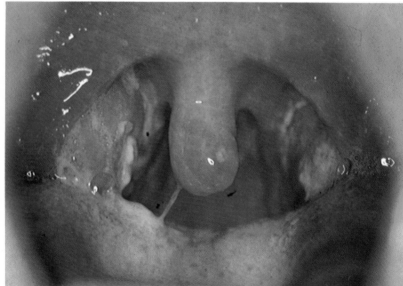

232

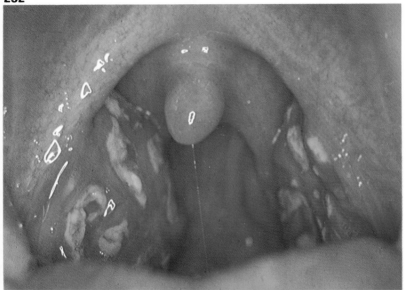

233

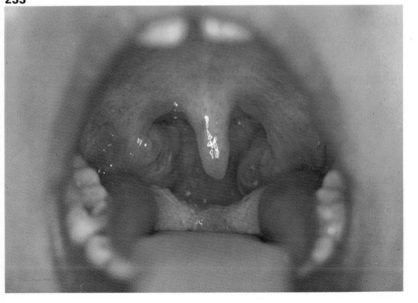

234   A quinsy   This is a complication of acute tonsillitis in which a peritonsillar abscess forms. The symptoms may be extremely severe with absolute dysphagia, pain referred to the ear and trismus. There is malaise, fever and marked swelling of the tonsillar lymph node. Examination shows the signs of acute tonsillitis with medial displacement of the tonsil to the midline.

If the abscess is pointing, incision at the site marked releases the pus. Since the advent of antibiotics the need for incision of quinsies is less. High doses of intramuscular penicillin for five days is the treatment and should be followed by a further five day course of oral penicillin. A large tonsil with medial displacement persists with inadequate treatment and represents a chronic quinsy in which recurrence of an acute episode is common. A throat swab of the pus is taken at the time of diagnosis and the result may later require the penicillin to be changed to another antibiotic.

A quinsy is extremely rare in children and is also rarely bilateral. Complications are uncommon, but *bleeding* from a quinsy is an important and serious sign : it is due to erosion by the peritonsillar pus of one of the adjacent vessels—either one of the tonsillar arteries or the internal carotid artery (bleeding quinsy). Quinsies not infrequently occur in those who have suffered previous episodes of acute tonsillitis. Tonsillectomy, which is indicated after a quinsy, is delayed four to six weeks until the acute phase has passed. Vascular fibrous tissue found lateral to the tonsil after a quinsy makes tonsillectomy technically difficult.

234

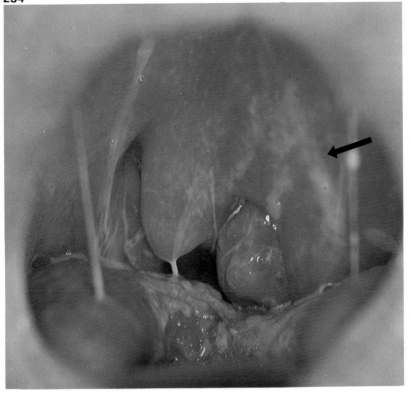

235 **Infectious mononucleosis** *This should be suspected if a sore throat persists despite antibiotic treatment, and a white cell analysis and Paul-Bunnell are indicated.* A white membrane covering one or both tonsils is characteristic and helpful in diagnosis. Hypersensitivity to ampicillin is increased with infectious mononucleosis, and this antibiotic should be avoided.

236 **Infectious mononucleosis in a patient without tonsils** In this case the membrane characteristic of infectious mononucleosis is seen either on the lingual tonsil or, as in this case, on a *prominent posterior pharyngeal band of lymphoid tissue.* A similar white membrane also covers the lymphoid tissue in the post-nasal space and the appearance on examination of the post-nasal space is suspicious of a neoplasm. The increase in bulk of the adenoids also causes a 'nasal voice', which is characteristic of infectious mononucleosis.

235

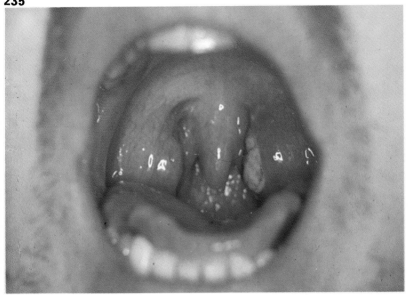

236

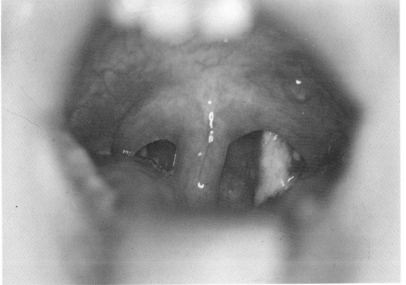

237 & 238   Monilia (thrush)   This is one of the fungal infections of the pharynx. Extensive white areas cover the entire oropharynx, and are not confined to the tonsil. The white areas are either continuous (**237**) or punctate (**238**). A swab confirms the diagnosis. The condition responds to antifungal mouth washes containing nystatin or amphotericin.

It is commoner in neonates than other age groups and may complicate treatment with broad spectrum antibiotics.

The extensive membrane (**237**) resembles diphtheria, but thrush is not usually associated with fever and toxaemia, and the membrane does not bleed on removal.

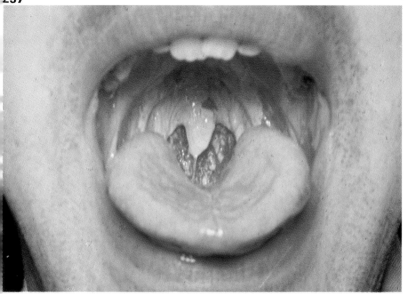

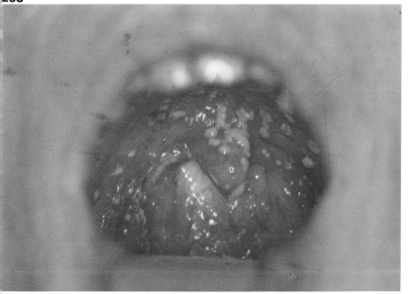

239   Chronic pharyngitis   In this condition there is a generalised hyperaemia of the pharyngeal mucous membrane, with hyperaemic masses of lymphoid tissue on the posterior wall of the oropharynx. A persistently slight sore throat is the main symptom. The cause is usually 'irritative' rather than due to chronic infection; environment and occupation, diet and tobacco are the common factors.

240   Scleroma with scarring of the soft palate and oropharynx
This is a specific chronic inflammatory disease of the upper respiratory tract mucosa predominantly occurring in Eastern Europe, Asia and South America. A protracted painless inflammation of the nose, pharynx, or larynx is followed after many years by extensive scarring, which is particularly apparent in the oropharynx. Unlike gummatous ulceration, which is a differential diagnosis, scleroma is not destructive, and the uvula is preserved, although it may be retracted by scarring into the naso-pharynx, and seen with the post-nasal mirror. The histology of the mucosa in scleroma is characteristic and diagnostic.

239

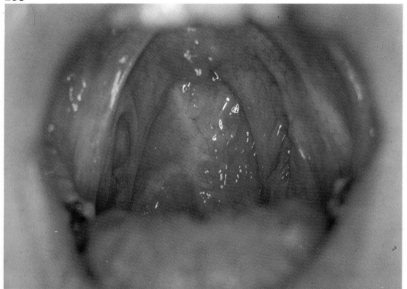

240

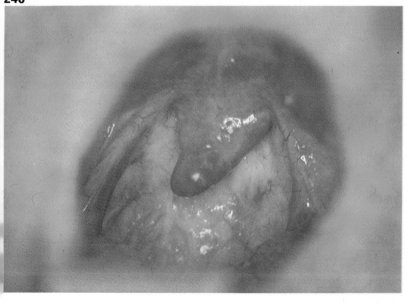

TONSILLECTOMY

This is the most frequently performed operation in the world. More strict indications for operating are, however, reducing the number of tonsillectomies. Recurrent episodes of acute tonsillitis, interfering with school or work, are the main indication: a quinsy or chronic tonsillitis are other indications.

241   The tonsillar fossae following tonsillectomy   These are covered with a white/yellow membrane for about ten days until the fossae are epithelialised.

242   Secondary infection   A blood clot in the tonsillar fossa is an important post-operative finding and almost certainly indicates secondary infection. This occurs between the third and tenth day and is associated with an increase in pain, and bleeding. The bleeding is usually scanty and settles when antibiotics control the secondary infection. Severe delayed bleeding after tonsillectomy may, however, occur, and the finding of a blood clot in a tonsillar fossa must not be ignored.

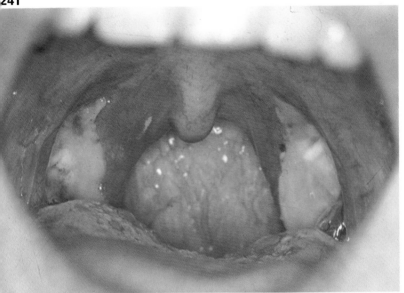

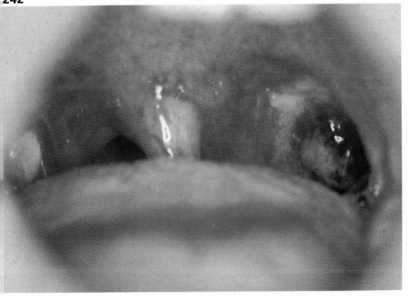

243 Bruising of the soft palate Such bruising and oedema of the uvula after tonsillectomy suggest unnecessary trauma at the time of operation. In this case there is also a clot in the tonsillar fossa—a sign of secondary infection.

244 Guillotine tonsillectomy Tonsillectomy today is by dissection with minimal injury to the fauces and surrounding structures. Adept use of the guillotine may also be a rapid and effective surgical technique, but removal of the uvula and fauces is possible in inexperienced hands. Fortunately *post-operative scarring* of the palate and uvula is frequently symptom-free.

243

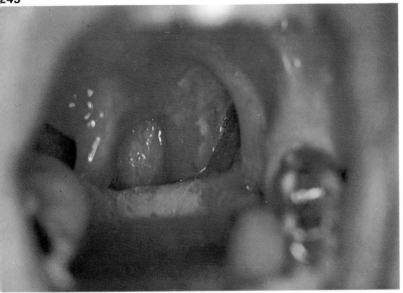

244

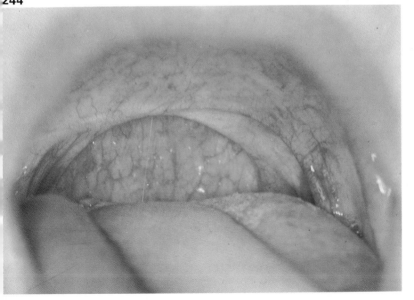

INFLAMMATION OF THE LARYNX

Laryngitis Whether acute or chronic, laryngitis presents with hoarseness and generalised hyperaemia of the laryngeal mucous membrane. Acute laryngitis commonly follows an upper respiratory tract infection, or is traumatic following vocal abuse. Voice rest is the most effective treatment. Chronic laryngitis may be associated with infection in the upper or lower respiratory tract, but is commonly irritative due to occupation and environment, vocal abuse or tobacco. The unusual laryngitis of myxoedema must also not be forgotten.

245 Normal vocal cords These are ivory coloured and smooth with few vessels on the surface. This is the view obtained through a laryngoscope at direct laryngoscopy.

246 Laryngeal nodules A specific and localised type of chronic laryngitis, seen in professional voice users, is *laryngeal nodules* (singers' nodes). Initially an oedema is seen on the vocal cord between the anterior one-third and posterior two-thirds of the cord. Later there is fibrin deposition beneath the squamous epithelium. Removal of the nodules may be necessary, but attention to the underlying voice production by a speech therapist is the most important aspect of treatment. These nodules are not an uncommon cause of *hoarseness in children*, particularly of large families involved in competitive shouting.

247 Juvenile papillomata is, however, the most important diagnosis to exclude in a hoarse child, for if the hoarseness is ignored stridor will develop as the papillomata extend to occlude the lumen of the larynx (as occurred in this post-mortem specimen).

In this curious condition multiple wart-like excrescences develop, usually before the age of five, on or around the vocal cords. Recurrence follows removal but fortunately there is regression or a reduced rate of growth at adolescence. The aetiology is unknown and the management is periodic microlaryngoscopy with meticulous removal of the papilloma to maintain an airway. A tracheostomy is avoided if possible for papillomata tend to develop on the tracheal opening. There is some evidence that ultrasound may be effective treatment, but radiotherapy is contra-indicated, as malignancy, normally not a complication, has developed in some cases following this treatment.

245

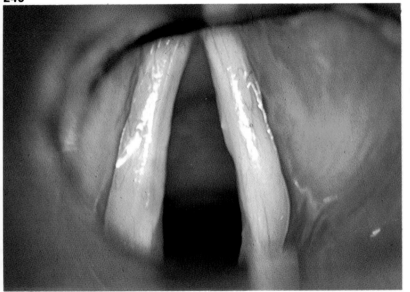

246

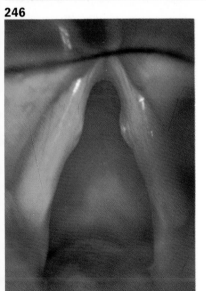

247

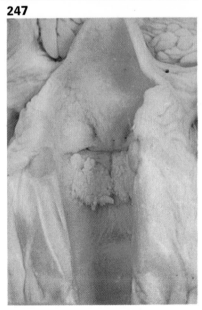

248 Singers' nodes with haemorrhage and oedema Singers' nodes are commonly bilateral and symmetrical, but haemorrhage and oedema can occur at the site of nodule formation after vocal abuse and may affect one cord.

249 Polypoid nodule A persistent polyp may result from such an episode. Established polypoid nodules or large nodules are not reversible and require surgical removal.

250 & 251 Large pedunculated polyp This may form on the vocal cord, and may be missed on examination, for it moves above and below the cord on expiration and inspiration. A large polyp in **250** is less apparent in **251** when it is below the cord on inspiration.

248

249

250

251

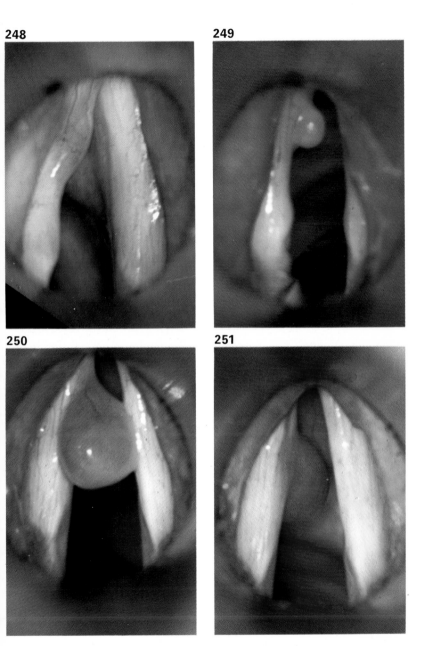

252 & 253   Intubation granulomas   These result from trauma by the anaesthetic tube to the vocal cord in the region of the vocal process of the arytenoid; they are therefore posterior. Removal at the pedicle is necessary but recurrence is not uncommon. **253** shows the pedicle of the intubation granuloma being held with forceps prior to removal.

254   Polyp at the anterior commissure   This is not always easy to see on indirect laryngoscopy for it may be partly obscured by the tubercle of the epiglottis. The laryngoscope is placed against the tubercle displacing it forwards and a clear view is obtained.

255   Haemangiomas   These are uncommon vocal cord lesions and if small may cause no hoarseness or bleeding, and be a chance finding on examination. Cryosurgery promises to be the most effective treatment for larger haemangiomas.

252

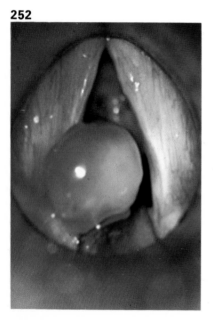

253

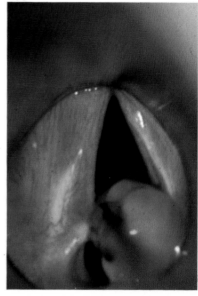

254

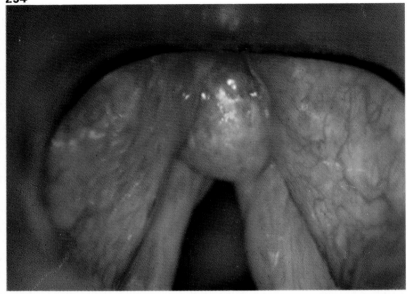

255

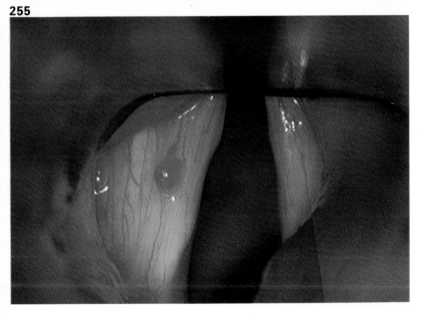

256 & 257   Chronic laryngitis   With this condition hyperaemia of the mucous membrane may be associated with other changes in the larynx. Oedema of the margin of the vocal cords is common, so that the free margin is polypoid (**256**) and a large sessile polyp may form (**257**). The oedema, although affecting both cords, may be more marked on one side.

Hypertrophy of the ventricular bands is another finding in chronic laryngitis, and they may meet in the midline on phonation producing a characteristic hoarseness.

258   Prolapse of the ventricular mucous membrane   This may also occur in chronic laryngitis and presents as a supraglottic swelling. A supraglottic cyst or carcinoma must be excluded.

259   Longstanding chronic laryngitis   The mucous membrane may become extremely hypertrophic with white patches (leucoplakia or hyperkeratosis). *Hyperkeratosis* is a premalignant condition. This patient had smoked over sixty cigarettes a day for fifty years.

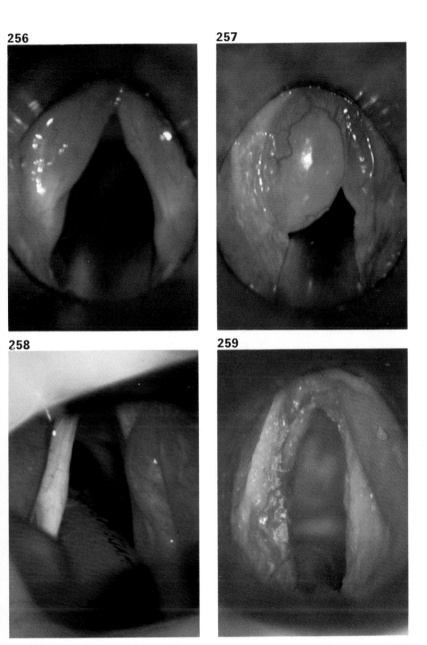

NEOPLASMS OF THE LARYNX

260   Carcinoma of the vocal cord   This usually occurs in smokers. The indurated leucoplakia on this vocal cord is a well differentiated squamous cell carcinoma that has arisen as a result of chronic laryngitis with hyperkeratosis. The prognosis for vocal cord carcinoma with radiotherapy is excellent, with a five year cure rate of over 90% for early lesions. The voice returns to normal, as does the appearance of the vocal cord.

261   Supraglottic squamous cell carcinoma   Carcinoma of the larynx commonly involves the vocal cord (glottic carcinoma), but lesions may develop below the cord (subglottic) or above the cord (supraglottic). The ulcerated area of granulation tissue above the oedematous vocal cord in this case is a squamous cell carcinoma. The prognosis for supraglottic and subglottic carcinoma is worse than for glottic carcinoma, for hoarseness is delayed until the cord is involved and the greater vascularity and lymphatic drainage above and below the cord predisposes to earlier metastasis.

260

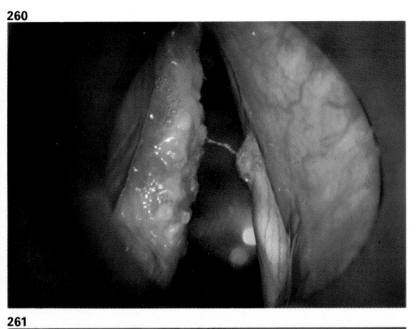

261

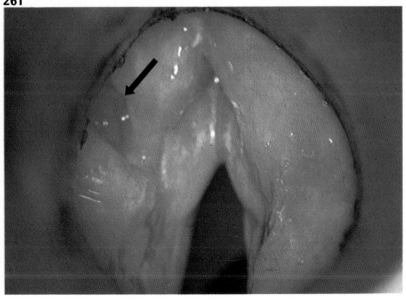

262   Total laryngectomy with left radical neck dissection
Nearly all cases of early carcinoma of the vocal cord are cured with radiotherapy. Disease, however, may remain with extensive cord carcinomas, with supra or subglottic lesions, or with carcinoma of the pyriform fossa or epiglottis. Partial laryngectomy (laryngofissure, extended laryngofissure or supraglottic laryngectomy) gives adequate resection of some laryngeal carcinomas, but frequently a total laryngectomy is required. This radical surgery, which may be associated with a neck dissection if the nodes are involved, means a permanent tracheostome, and an alternative method of speech has to be developed. Air is swallowed into the upper oesophagus and coherent speech is achieved by learning to phonate with controlled regurgitation of the air.

A radical neck dissection (or block dissection) involves removal of the superficial and deep cervical lymph nodes from the anterior and posterior triangles of the neck. To ensure removal of these nodes necessitates removal of the sterno-mastoid, digastric and omohyoid muscles along with the submandibular gland and internal jugular vein. Despite this extensive removal of neck tissue, post-operative disability is limited to a shoulder weakness, for the accessory cranial nerve which supplies the trapezius muscle, is divided during a neck dissection.

263   Stomal stud   Stenosis of the tracheostome is sometimes a post-operative problem and a small stomal stud can be used by the patient.

264   Laryngectomy specimen   This specimen has a large supraglottic carcinoma and shows the hyoid, thyroid and cricoid cartilages and upper rings of trachea, which are removed at laryngectomy.

262

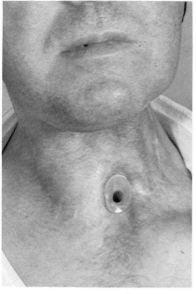

263

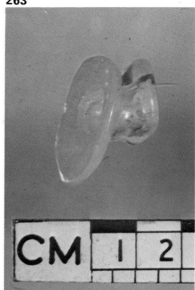

264

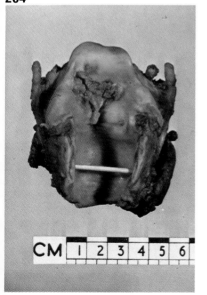

265   Laryngeal tomogram of a fibroma   The laryngeal tomogram (on page 38) is a helpful investigation for a larynx that is difficult or impossible to see on indirect examination. This tomogram shows a large pedunculated supraglottic swelling, which proved to be a fibroma—a rare benign laryngeal tumour.

266   Secondaries from lung carcinoma   Hoarseness may be due to *paralysis of one vocal cord.* Lack of cord movement on phonation is diagnosed on indirect laryngoscopy. Although temporary idiopathic cord palsy is the single most common cause, involvement of the left recurrent laryngeal nerve in chest disease must be excluded. Any hilar lymph node lesion in the region of the aortic arch may involve this nerve, such as secondaries from lung carcinoma. The enlarged left atrium of mitral stenosis may also press on the left recurrent laryngeal nerve and cause hoarseness, as may an aortc aneurysm or the enlarged pulmonary artery of pulmonary hypertension.

The recurrent laryngeal nerves are also occasionally damaged in the neck by severe external injury, or by thyroid carcinoma or by thyroid surgery. Central lesions, or lesions near the jugular foramen involving the vagus may also cause cord paralysis, and hoarseness is one of the symptoms of posterior inferior cerebellar artery thrombosis.

Hoarseness, particularly a whispered voice, with a normal larynx is probably a functional voice problem. *Hysterical aphonia* is not uncommon in young women, and stems from a superficial psychiatric upset. Treatment from the speech therapist is usually effective without referral to a psychiatrist being necessary. Curious alterations in the voice or hoarseness may also be due to a hysterical dysphonia.

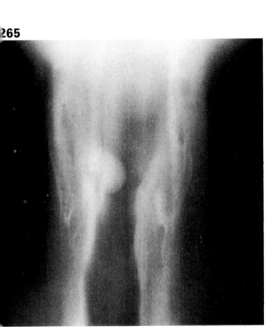

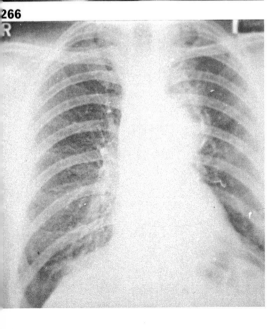

MICROSURGERY OF THE LARYNX

267   Operating microscope   The use of the microscope for direct laryngoscopy has greatly increased the scope and precision of laryngeal surgery. All small benign lesions of the larynx are better excised with this technique. Biopsies of malignant disease can be accurately taken from the suspicious area with minimal damage to adjacent tissue.

268   The holder for the laryngoscope rests on the patient's chest and enables the surgeon to have both hands free for instrumentation. The patient's x-rays are seen in the background: the chest x-ray and x-ray of the cervical spine are routine investigations before direct laryngoscopy.

Cold light instruments give brighter and more reliable illumination than bulbs, and the development of a light transmitting glass fibre cable has been another advance in endoscopy.

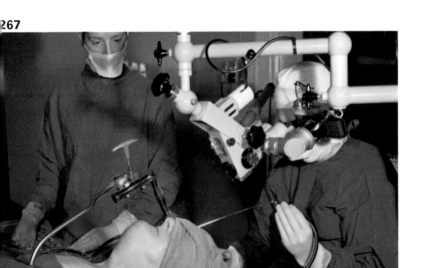

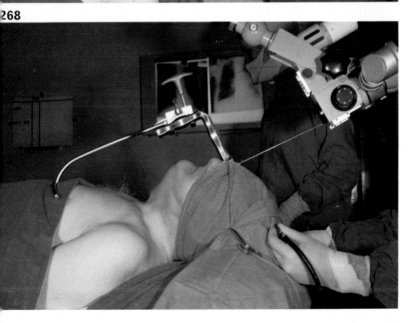

TRACHEOSTOMY

269 A patient after tracheostomy   Obstruction of the larynx causes stridor and may necessitate a tracheostomy. Acute inflammatory conditions of the upper respiratory tract e.g. epiglottitis, or foreign bodies or neoplasms limiting the airway are the commonest causes of stridor.

Tracheostomy is also required for respiratory failure due to central depression of the respiratory centre e.g. strokes, barbiturate poisoning or head injury. Also, if the efferent nerves to the muscles of respiration are damaged, e.g. poliomyelitis, tetanus. Multiple rib fractures or severe chest infections may require tracheostomy. Tracheostomy enables breathing to be controlled by an intermittent positive pressure respirator, and bronchial secretions can be removed with suction. A prolonged obstruction of the glottis may occur with juvenile papillomata, severe trauma to the larynx, or with bilateral cord palsies, and a permanent tracheostomy is necessary. A tracheostomy tube with a *speaking valve* allows air to enter during inspiration but closes on expiration so that air passes through the larynx for phonation.

Emergency tracheostomy may be a difficult operation, particularly under local anaesthetic when a general anaesthetic with intubation is not practical. An opening into the trachea through the cricothyroid membrane offers a simpler and more direct relief for upper respiratory tract obstruction.

270 Cricothyreotomy cannula with trocar   This instrument has been devised for emergency operations. A tracheostomy can later be performed when the emergency of the acute obstruction is past.

269

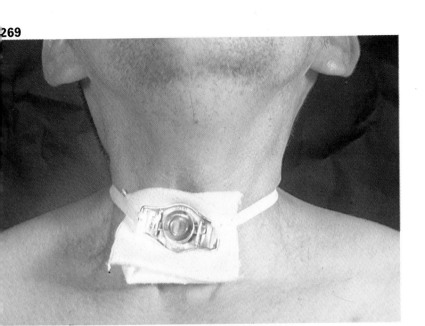

270

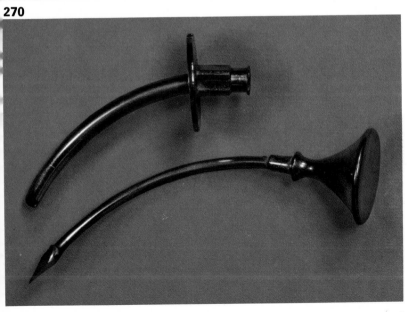

THE HYPOPHARYNX AND OESOPHAGUS

271   Globus pharyngeus   This is a common condition in which the patient, usually a young girl, complains of a sensation of a lump in the throat. The site indicated is the cricoid region. In the history a helpful direct question is to ask whether the lump is most apparent on swallowing food, fluid or saliva: the patient with globus will consistently reply that saliva is the problem, and that the symptom occurs *between* meals.

272   Barium swallow   Globus pharyngeus is a psychosomatic condition but there is demonstrable spasm of the cricopharyngeus on barium swallow, where the barium column is seen to be 'nipped'. Over-attention and concern by the patient perpetuates the spasm and reassurance is usually the only treatment required.

Globus pharyngeus does not necessarily occur in hysterics and globus hystericus is a misnomer. It is also a condition that calls for investigation, particularly in the older age group. when it may be the presenting symptom of disease in the oesophagus or stomach. Hiatus hernia and oesophageal reflux commonly cause cricopharyngeal spasm, and gastric ulcers and neoplasms may also present with globus. A barium swallow and meal is therefore an important investigation. Cervical osteoarthritis with marked changes in the region of the 6th cervical vertebra may also give rise to globus.

271

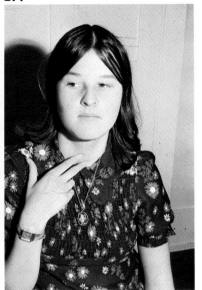

272

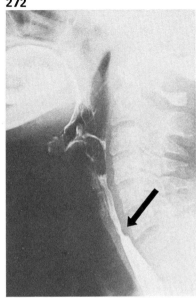

273 & 274   Pharyngeal pouch   This is a herniation of mucous membrane through the posterior fibres of the inferior constrictor above the cricopharyngeus, usually occurring in old age. The defect predisposing to its development is a failure of co-ordinated relaxation of the cricopharyngeus on swallowing. A pouch is frequently associated with hiatus hernia.

A small pouch causes no symptoms but, when large, dysphagia, varying from slight to absolute, develops. There is regurgitation of undigested food, and gurgling may be heard in the neck after eating, or a swelling may be seen, laterally in the neck, usually on the left.

The pouch accumulates food, and spill into the respiratory tract may cause coughing. A pouch may in fact present with respiratory disease, either a bronchitis, or apical fibrosis simulating tuberculosis, or as acute pulmonary infection—either a bronchitis, a bronchopneumonia or a lung abscess.

The Barium swallow is the only investigation required to confirm the diagnosis of a pharyngeal pouch.

If symptoms are marked, excision of the pouch via a neck incision is necessary. Rarely a carcinoma occurs within the lumen of a pharyngeal pouch.

273

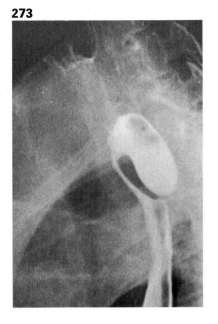

274

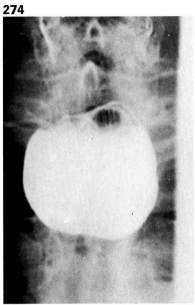

275–278   Foreign bodies in the oesophagus   Foreign bodies such as bones (**275**), coins (**276**), pins (**277**), dentures and small toys, may impact in the upper third of the oesophagus. A history of possible foreign impaction must not be ignored for oesophageal perforation leads to cervical cellulitis and mediastinitis, which may be fatal. Air seen on x-ray behind the pharynx and oesophagus is diagnostic of a perforation (**278**). Persistent dysphagia, pain referred to the neck or back, pain on inspiration and fever all suggest a foreign body. Chest x-ray and x-ray of the neck are essential investigations, but even if negative, persistent symptoms are suspicious and oesophagoscopy is necessary.

Coins, however, which pass the cricopharyngeus usually traverse the rest of the gut, and rarely require removal.

275

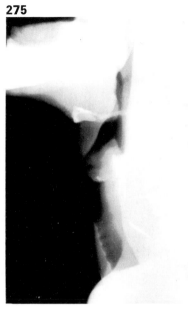

276

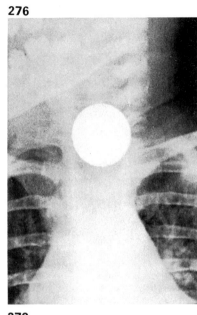

277

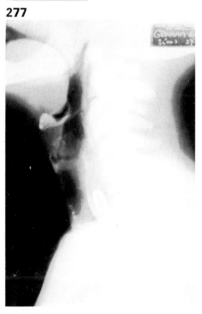

278

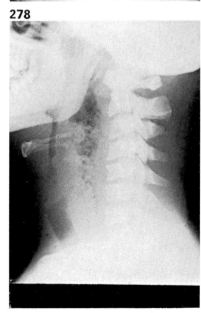

279 & 280   Carcinoma of the pyriform fossa and upper oesophagus   The presenting signs are dysphagia for solids, and pain, commonly referred to the ear. There is early metastasis to the cervical nodes. A carcinoma involving mainly the medial wall of the pyriform fossa causes hoarseness. The prognosis is not good, particularly with upper oesophageal carcinoma, whether treatment is with radiotherapy or surgery. Resection involves a pharyngolaryngectomy, and the replacement or reconstruction of the cervical oesophagus poses major technical problems. Immediate replacement with stomach (or colon) mobilised and brought through the thorax and sutured to the pharynx are current techniques. The delayed use of neck and chest skin flaps is an alternative method of reconstruction (**280**).

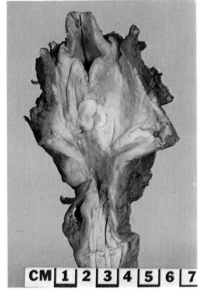

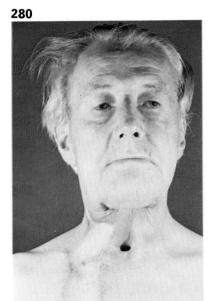

The Head and Neck

SALIVARY GLANDS

281 Submandibular calculus A calculus obstructing the sub-mandibular duct causes painful and intermittent enlargement of the gland. The swelling occurs on eating and regresses slowly : secondary infection in the gland leads to persistent tender swelling of the gland.

The swelling in the submandibular triangle is visible and palpable bimanually, with one finger in the mouth.

282 Grossly enlarged gland This develops if an impacted calculus is ignored. A neoplasm of the submandibular gland is the differential diagnosis if the enlargement is persistent. Mumps may also cause a tender submandibular gland swelling, and an enlarged lymph node in the submandibular triangle, frequently secondary to dental infection, simulates gland involvement.

283 X-ray of submandibular gland The calculi show clearly. in the duct.

284 Calculus impacted in the gland If the calculus is in the duct, removal by intra-oral incision is effective. If, however, the calculus is placed posteriorly in the duct or is impacted in the gland (as here) excision of the submandibular gland is required. Care is taken in this operation to preserve the mandibular branch of the facial nerve which crosses the submandibular triangle to supply the muscles of the angle of the mouth.

281

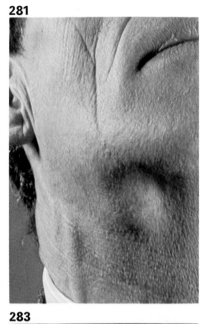

282

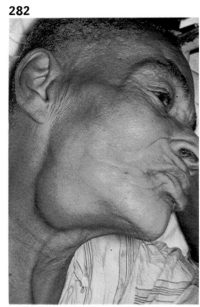

283

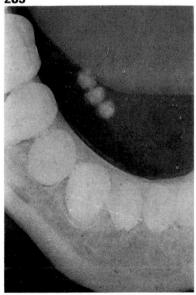

284

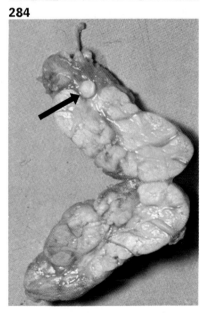

285 & 286   Mixed parotid tumour (pleomorphic adenoma)
These present as a firm smooth non-tender swelling. The growth is slow so the history may be long. The bulk of the parotid gland lies in the *neck* posterior to the ramus of the mandible, and parotid tumours do not usually cause swelling on the face.

287   Sebaceous cyst   A swelling in the parotid region, but on the face suggests another diagnosis: there is a small punctum on the swelling in this picture, diagnostic of a sebaceous cyst.

288   Congenital hypertrophy of the masseter muscle   Careful palpation follows observation of a swelling, and what appears as a parotid mass here is palpable as a congenital hypertrophy of the masseter muscle.

A softer swelling in the tail of the parotid may be an *adenolymphoma*, a benign tumour of salivary gland tissue within a parotid lymph node.

The pleomorphic adenoma is a low-grade malignant tumour, and is commonly in the superficial lobe of the parotid: treatment is superficial parotidectomy with preservation of the facial nerve. A soft parotid swelling with a short history and a partial or complete facial palsy is probably a cylindroma or carcinoma, requiring total parotidectomy with sacrifice of the facial nerve, and radiotherapy.

285

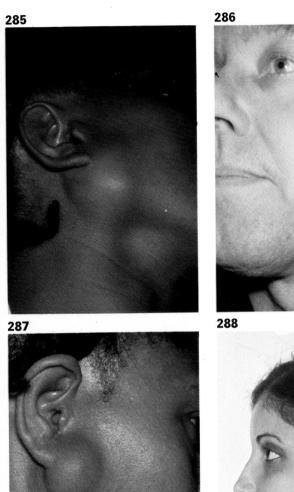

286

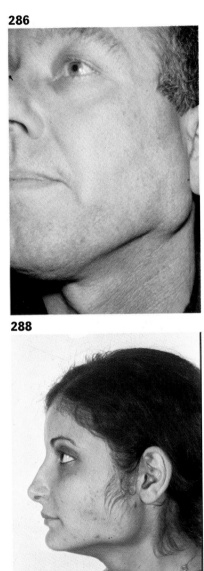

287

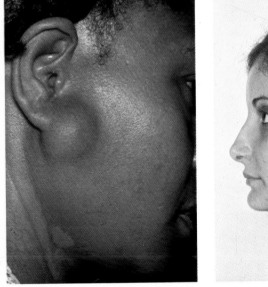

288

289 Sialectasis of the parotid gland This presents as inter-mittent episodes of painful swelling. Calculi in the parotid duct are uncommon and are not easily demonstrated on x-ray. An intraoral view is necessary. A sialogram confirms sialectasis, and the punctate dilations of the parotid ducts are similar in appearance to bronchiectasis.

290 Normal submandibular sialogram The pattern of ducts not involved with sialectasis is demonstrated.

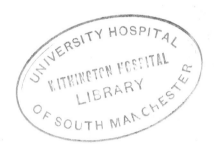

UNIVERSITY HOSPITAL
WITHINGTON HOSPITAL
LIBRARY
OF SOUTH MANCHESTER

289

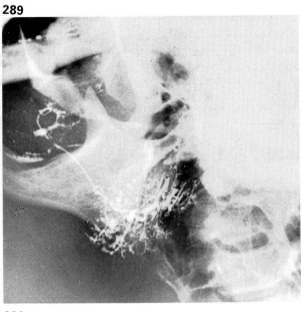

290

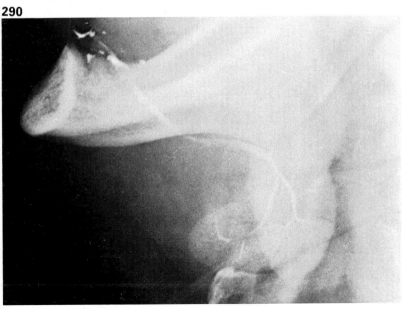

INFLAMMATORY NECK SWELLINGS

Spread of dental infection must be remembered as a possible cause of inflammatory neck swelling.

291   Ludwig's angina   An indurated tender *midline* inflammation is characteristic of Ludwig's angina. Bimanual palpation reveals a characteristic woody firmness of the normally soft tissues of the floor of the mouth and this is an early sign. This acute infection may spread from the apices of the lower incisors and in this case followed extraction. In the pre-antibiotic era this condition was serious because spread of infection involved the larynx, and caused the acute onset of stridor. This complication is still to be remembered although extensive neck incisions to relieve pus under pressure are rarely necessary, and the response to intramuscular penicillin is good.

292   Extensive cervical cellulitis   This may develop from a dental abscess in the lower molars, and involves the neck laterally.

293   Submental sinus   A chronic localised midline infection under the chin is probably a submental sinus. This recurrent mass of granulation tissue formed at the opening of a sinus leading to apical infection in a lower incisor.

294   Tuberculous cervical abscesses   These are uncommon in countries where cattle are tuberculin tested, for intake of infected milk is the usual cause. A chronic discharging neck abscess in the posterior triangle is characteristic of tuberculosis. Firm, non-tender nodes without sinus formation in the same site are also suggestive of tuberculosis. Chemotherapy alone usually fails to control this condition and excision of the nodes or chronic abscesses is required.

291

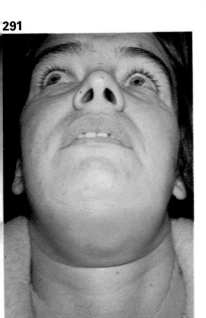

292

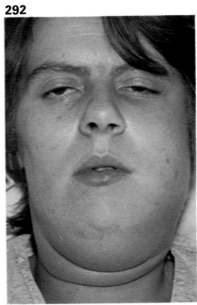

293

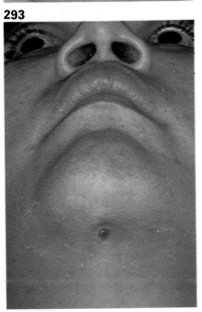

294

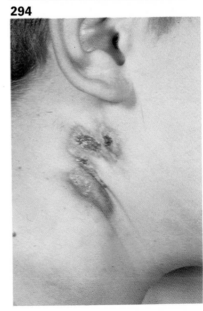

MIDLINE NECK SWELLINGS

295 & 296   Thyroglossal cyst   This is a midline neck swelling forming in the remnant of the thyroglossal tract. The swelling is commonly between the thyroid and hyoid but suprahyoid cysts also occur. The convexity of the hyoid bone and thyroid cartilage push the cyst to one side so it may not be strictly midline. The cyst moves on swallowing and on protrusion of the tongue. It may be non-tender or present with recurrent episodes of acute swelling and tenderness. Treatment is excision with removal of the body of the hyoid bone. Failure to excise the body of the hyoid predisposes to recurrence for the thyro-glossal tract extends in a loop deep to the hyoid bone.

297 & 298   Dermoids   Midline neck swellings in the submandibular region (**297**) or suprasternal region (**298**) are commonly dermoids.

295

296

297

298

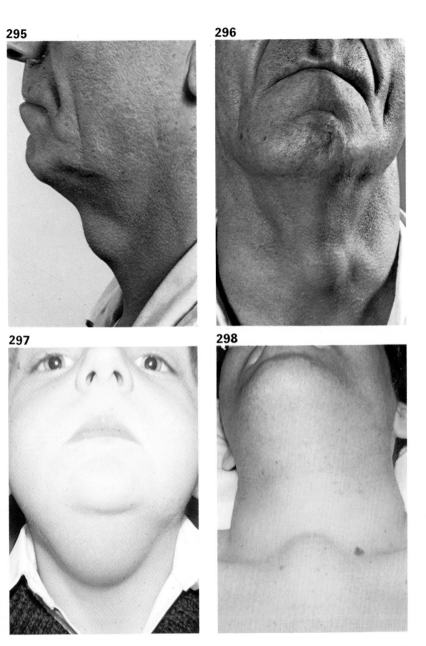

LATERAL NECK SWELLINGS

299 & 300   Branchial cyst   This has a consistent site, is smooth and, if there is no secondary infection, is non-tender. It lies between the upper one-third and lower two-thirds of the anterior border of the sternomastoid and is deep to and partly concealed by this muscle. The cyst can therefore be large by the time it presents. When excised the deep surface is found to be closely related to the internal jugular vein.

A metastatic lymph node from the thyroid, upper respiratory tract (e.g. nasopharynx), or post-cricoid region, and swellings of neurogenous origin (chemodectomas, neurofibromas, neuroblastomas) are among the important differential diagnoses of a lateral neck swelling. The ubiquitous lipoma is also not uncommon in the neck, and in children the cystic hygroma is to be remembered. Hodgkin's disease also frequently presents with an enlarged cervical lymph node.

301   Laryngocele   This is an unusual neck swelling that the patient can inflate with the Valsalva manoeuvre. It is an enlargement of the laryngeal ventricle into the neck between the hyoid and thyroid cartilage. It tends to occur in musicians who play wind instruments, or glass blowers. A laryngocele can become infected and present as a pyolaryngocele, causing obstruction to the airway.

299

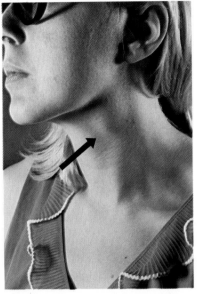

300

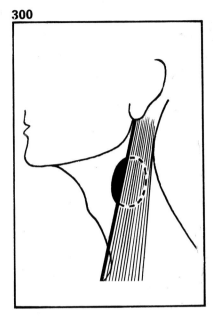

301

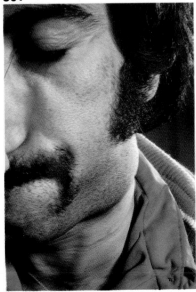

233

302 Horner's Syndrome Pressure on the sympathetic nerve trunk in the neck, particularly by malignant disease, causes changes in the eye. Ptosis, with a small pupil, is apparent in the patient's left eye: this is also associated with an enophthalmos and a lack of sweating. With a cervical swelling examination should exclude Horner's syndrome.

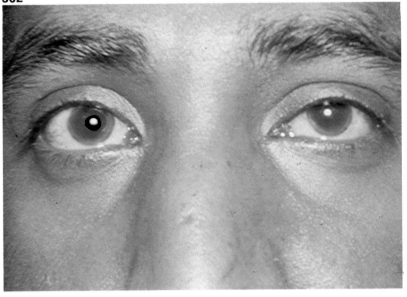

INDEX